More praise for *Rainforest Home Remedies*

"A stimulating, information-filled, and well-organized account of the main features of contemporary Maya folk medicine."

—Michael Harner, Ph.D., author of *The Way of the Shaman*

"Our disconnection from nature is a serious cause of illness. Rosita Arvigo and Nadine Epstein help us to remember our connection with plants that can heal us as the authors bring us back home to a sacred way of life."

—Sandra Ingerman, author of *Soul Retrieval* and *Medicine for the Earth*

"Dr. Arvigo has been a conscientious student of her Maya teachers for nearly two decades. This book is a magnificent tribute to her teachers, providing useful information for all of us. The remedies are explained in a simple but comprehensive fashion, using plants that can be easily found. . . . A wonderful compilation of fascinating reading."

—Michael J. Balick, Ph.D., director and philecology curator of economic botany, Institute of Economic Botany, The New York Botanical Garden

"Thank you for bringing these precious thoughts, so comprehensively done, to the healing world. If we are to survive as a species, it will be because ideas like these become important again."

—Patch Adams, M.D., author of *Gesundheit!*

"Two great modern mothers introduce you to the best of old (pre-Columbian) Mayan and new (European introduction) Mayan medicine, a practical blend of the old and the new."

—James Duke, Ph.D., author of *The Green Pharmacy*

"A practical guide to healthy living and traditional herbal wisdom, blended artfully with an insightful view of common modern ailments. Full of stories; a refreshing view of wellness and sane living that is so needed today."

—Christopher Hobbs, fourth-generation herbalist and author of *Herbal Remedies for Dummies*

RAINFOREST HOME REMEDIES

The Maya Way to Heal Your Body
& Replenish Your Soul

ROSITA ARVIGO
& NADINE EPSTEIN

HarperSanFrancisco
A Division of HarperCollins Publishers

HarperCollins books may be purchased for educational, business, or sales promotional use. For information please write: Special Markets Department, HarperCollins Publishers, 10 East 53rd Street, New York, NY 10022.

HarperCollins Web site: http://www.harpercollins.com

HarperCollins®, 📖 ®, and HarperSanFrancisco™ are trademarks of Harper-Collins Publishers, Inc.

FIRST EDITION

Library of Congress Cataloging-in-Publication Data

Arvigo, Rosita.
    Rainforest home remedies : the Maya way to heal your body and replenish your soul / Rosita Arvigo and Nadine Epstein.
        p.   cm.
    Includes bibliographical references and index.
    ISBN 0–06–251637-X (paper)
        1. Alternative medicine. 2. Mayas—Medicine. 3. Traditional medicine.
4. Rain forest ecology. 5. Medicinal plants. I. Epstein, Nadine. II. Title.
R733.A75 2001
615.8'82'0972824—dc21   00-040878

01 02 03 04 05 ❖/RRD(H) 10 9 8 7 6 5 4 3 2 1

This book is written in memory of Don Elijio Panti
and other traditional healers.

They are the "ones who know" and who hold fast to the
truth through difficult times.

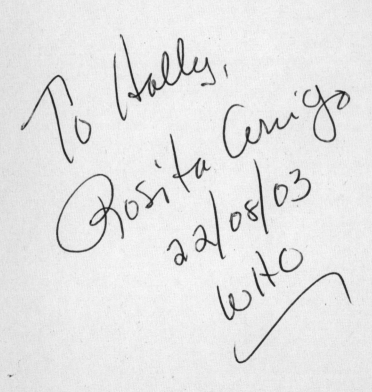

This book was a joint project, but because most of the professional and personal experiences related are those of Rosita Arvigo, we chose to write some sections in the first-person voice.

Contents

Preface: What Maya Healing Can Do for You!   ix
Prologue   xi

PART I
Introduction to Maya Medicine   1

PART II
Physical Ailments   41
 General Ailments of Adults   44
 Physical Ailments of Women   90
 Physical Ailments of Men   109
 Physical Ailments of Infants and Children   114

PART III
Maya Bodywork and Massage   129

PART IV
Maya Spiritual Illness and Healing   151

PART V
Maya Daily Wisdom: Nine Pointers for Healthy Living   191

Acknowledgments   197
Latin Names of Plants   203
Resources   205
Bibliography   213
Index   215

What Maya Healing Can Do for You!

Why should you use the remedies and information in this book instead of depending on what our society considers "traditional"—the triumvirate of Tylenol, Prozac, and Viagra? Why should a harried and hurried person like you make time for Maya healing?

As you will see in this book, Maya healing

- Addresses about 85 percent of common ailments
- Puts you more in control of your own healing process
- Reestablishes and deepens your sense of connection to the natural world
- Expands your team of healing helpers by teaching you to call upon plants, massage, bathing, prayers, and rituals
- Allows room for the unknown and the unseen, both within and without
- Adds a spiritual component to healing that is mostly missing from modern medicine
- Adds the idea of humans as energy beings to our thinking about healing, a notion long maintained by many ancient peoples, including Native Americans, Indians, and Chinese, and now supported by research
- Demonstrates that investing time in healing is fulfilling
- Deepens your understanding of the world

- Teaches you that nature is not frightening and unknowable
- Allows you to try natural, nontoxic, and inexpensive alternatives that complement modern medicine
- Helps to build community by encouraging people to help others
- Leads to longer-lasting healing
- Strengthens the body and soul rather than weakening them
- Considers your soul as part of the picture
- Encourages a spiritual view of our world, increasing awareness
- Explains misunderstood human suffering
- Works in harmony with your body's natural inclination to heal itself

Finally, Maya healing is enjoyable. There's nothing much lovelier than a Maya spiritual bath created with plants, loving intent, and prayer.

So why not learn from the Maya? Take the best of true traditional wisdom and apply it to your own harried life. Try it, and see what Maya healing can do for you.

Prologue

Don Elijio Panti, one of the last great Maya *h'mens*, died in 1996 at the age of 103. *H'men* (heh-men) means "one who knows" in Mopan Maya. The h'men is the doctor-priest or priestess who has the ability to heal in both the physical and spiritual realms.

Don Elijio was born in San Andreas, a small Mopan Maya village on a steep slope rising from Lake Peten Itza in Peten, Guatemala. When he was eleven months old, his father got drunk and killed a man. Don Elijio's mother wrapped her son in her *reboso* and fled with her husband across the border to neighboring Belize, then British Honduras.

Don Elijio grew up in the charming riverside Maya village of Succotz, a few kilometers from Belize's western border with Guatemala. His youth was dominated by his father, a well-known *hechisero*—a person who practices evil magic and uses his powers to hurt rather than to heal.

Although the young Elijio had a natural affinity for plants and healing, he wanted nothing to do with his father's path. Like many men of his time, he married young—at fifteen—and went to work to support his family as a *chiclero*. For months at a time he lived and worked in chicle camps deep in the rainforest. Until synthetic gum was developed in the 1930s, chicle was the main ingredient of chewing gum. The chicle sap was laboriously extracted from the sapodilla tree. It was tough and dangerous work. When the camps closed, the men and women who made their living there were forced to find new lines of work.

During Don Elijio's last season as a chiclero he worked in a camp near the ruins of the Maya city of Tikal in Guatemala. There he met Jeronimo Requena, the bush doctor for the camp and a powerful h'men. Don Elijio needed a new profession, and Requena took it upon himself to train Don Elijio in the healing arts.

So it came to pass that Don Elijio became a student of an oral tradition that had been passed from h'men to h'men for thousands of years. He learned in the shadow of the great Temple of the Jaguar at Tikal. He was about thirty years old at the time.

After two years of learning about medicinal plants and praying to the Maya spirits, Don Elijio received his *sastun*. A sastun is a stone or crystal that some healers use to communicate with the spirit world. His was a greenish, translucent stone about the size of a marble. Possession of the sastun marked him as a h'men.

Don Elijio spent most of the next six decades dispensing healing wisdom out of his tiny, ramshackle clinic in the small Maya village of San Antonio, located in the foothills of the Maya Mountains. San Antonio had a long history of shamans and initiate training.[1] Don Elijio focused his practice on medicinal plants, bodywork, and physical and spiritual healing. His reputation grew. Although San Antonio wasn't easy to reach, people in need made it to his clinic by foot and mule, and later by car and pickup truck.

Life wasn't easy for Don Elijio. Like most traditional healers, he never made much money. Nor was he always given the respect he was due. In the 1950s, when Protestant evangelism swept through Central America, many villagers converted, including some of Don Elijio's grandchildren with whom he lived. Although his clinic was rarely empty, he was dismissed by many as a relic from the past who dispensed worthless superstitions. Some villagers even accused him of being an evil magician.

Such accusations were not new to the Maya. From the moment the Spanish came ashore in the 1500s, Maya beliefs had been belittled. The Spanish called the Maya h'mens *brujos,* or witches, and the first bishop of Yucatan, Father Diego de Landa, called the Maya "demon worshipers." Despite the oppression, the Maya held on to much of their religion, incorporating their own beliefs into Catholicism. Over time the Catholic Church grew comfortably tolerant of Maya beliefs. The evangelists are less tolerant.

Interestingly enough, medical doctors and nurses in Belize did not ostracize Don Elijio and occasionally even referred difficult cases to him. Modern-day Belize, with a population of less than two hundred thousand, is a multilingual, multiethnic community accustomed to different cultural and medical practices. For generations villagers depended on traditional healers, who were respected members of the community. As a result, allopathic medicine has never achieved the exclusive dominance in Belize that it has in the United States and Europe.

When I first met Don Elijio in 1982, it was at a low point in his life. He was in his eighties, and no one was seriously interested in learning the old ways. Traditionally Maya h'mens pass their knowledge to chosen apprentices. Don Elijio had no apprentice.

Chinda, his wife of sixty-five years, had died, and he was achingly lonely. He was remarkably healthy, except for a fondness for the bottle. For three years following Chinda's death he drank steadily, drowning his pain and nearly killing himself. By the time I showed up in San Antonio he had stopped drinking.

When I saw that he had no apprentice, I volunteered. He refused my offer.

"It would do no good to teach a *gringa*," he explained. "You must go home one day, it is only natural, and what I taught you would be lost up there."

I spent a year as his assistant, working hard to prove myself. I did my best to make myself useful. I chopped plants and picked corn, spent countless hours listening to his wonderful stories, and used my skills as a massage therapist to ease his aches. Eventually he relented and agreed to teach me, on the condition that I would never leave his people without a healer. I agreed.

I was fortunate to have a husband and family who supported me through the ten years of training that followed. During this time Don Elijio and I became very close friends. He referred to me as his daughter.

Since the story of my years with Don Elijio, *Sastun: My Apprenticeship with a Maya Healer*, was published in 1994, I have received thousands of letters, e-mails, and phone calls from people intrigued by the possibilities of Maya medicine. Many wrote to express their thrill at having the opportunity to meet Don Elijio through the book. They said that the book had made them feel as if they were actually right there with us in the rainforest. Thousands have visited the rainforest medicine trail at Ix Chel Farm in Belize. Many more have attended my workshops and lectures around the world. And every day I receive a letter, call, e-mail, or visit from someone in search of a cure for themselves or a loved one.

To be honest, the attention has been rather overwhelming, and I have struggled with what Don Elijio warned me would be my fate. Traditionally Maya healers are both exalted and debased by the people they help.

"This is a lonely road, my child," Don Elijio used to tell me. "*Curanderos* [ones who cure] are not often trusted by the very people they heal. They fear us, they envy us, and some hate us. The gossip never ends. When we heal people who couldn't find help elsewhere, they call us witches. Then at night, when you drop your weary body in the hammock, you hear *knock-knock,* and there is the person who called you a witch holding an infant on the doorstep of death. There is no rest by day or night."

It has come to pass just as he warned. Privacy is difficult to find, and I am often the focus of envy and suspicion. Time too has become a precious and elusive commodity.

I find that I can turn away no one who is in need and at the same time I cannot personally meet with everyone. Nor is it possible to respond to all those who write seeking help. Don Elijio may have had a constant stream of patients at his door, but he didn't have a phone, an e-mail address, a fax machine, or a post office box, and he didn't travel the world.

This book is the solution to this dilemma: it is for those who want to learn and incorporate the healing knowledge of the ancient Maya into their personal and professional lives but do not have the time or opportunity to study in person with a great teacher.

Writing down what I have learned from Don Elijio and other traditional healers over the past twenty years feels more crucial since Don Elijio's death. He lapsed into his final illness in 1996. Although he was impressively strong of body and mind until about a year before he died, his descent into death was difficult. His last days were painful to watch.

In death Don Elijio was showered with the recognition he had long deserved. Hundreds of deeply grateful patients attended an impressive state funeral. Dignitaries, neighbors, and professors eulogized this humble man who had given the world so much of his love, humor, warmth, and healing. Some of the same people who had ridiculed him as a relic, a fool, and a demon worshiper also came to praise him.

One night I even received a call on our crackling radiophone in Belize from a kind reporter from the *New York Times.* He was writing an obituary of Don Elijio, who had never been to the United States and had rarely traveled more than fifty miles from San Antonio. He was illiterate and had never read a newspaper in his life. He had never heard of the *New York Times.*

The headline of the obituary read: "Maya Healer with Modern Ties." The reporter went on to say:

Elijio Panti, a traditional healer whose ancient herbal remedies attracted the attention of modern medical scientists and drew thousands of patients to the door of his humble hut in Belize, died on Sunday in his home in the village of San Antonio. He was 103 and widely regarded as the last Maya master healer in Belize.

The night of Don Elijio's death, my husband, Greg, had a dream. In the dream I was in bed and Don Elijio was lying on the floor. He looked old and sick. Suddenly he rose up and was transformed into a young, stronger Don Elijio. He got into bed, gave me a kiss and a hug, and gestured with his hand to the corner of the room. There in the corner was a Maya boy of about fifteen. The boy's face continually transformed into the faces of other Maya boys and girls.

Don Elijio then said: "Take the children as though they were your own. Train them and teach them to help each other."

In honor of his last request, Ix Chel Farm holds a ten-day summer camp that teaches children the importance of conserving medicinal plants and preserving traditional healing. Traditional healers are on hand daily to tell stories, share knowledge, and demonstrate the uses of their healing tools. It is our hope that one of these campers will someday become a h'men and continue the unbroken chain of knowledge.

How to Use This Book

The Maya have so much to teach us!

This is a self-help book based on the principles of Maya medicine and Maya healing wisdom. You will find easy-to-follow, time-honored instructions for the preparation of ancient and contemporary remedies that will assist your body's natural capacity to be self-regulating, self-healing, and self-regenerating. This book also provides time-honored instructions for a healthy soul and spirit.

Some Maya remedies cannot be undertaken without the personal guidance of a h'men, but we have included here the many that you can use on your own. This book will not teach you how to become a h'men. It does, however, speak to the most important function of a h'men—true healing.

Important Maya Healing Terms

H'men (heh-men): one who knows, healer, doctor-priest, shaman

Ch'ulel (ch-oo-lel): the life force that permeates all of existence; similar to the Chinese *chi* or Indian *prahna*

Sastun (sas-toon): stone or crystal used by a h'men to communicate with the Maya spirits

Xiv (sheev): medicinal plants

Whatever your interest, the rest of the book will make much more sense if you start by reading the introduction. There you will become familiar with the Maya approach to healing, the roots of Maya healing wisdom, and the Maya worldview.

Part II explains remedies for common physical ailments and includes sections on the ailments unique to women, men, and children. All ailments are arranged alphabetically for easy reference.

As you will see, the Maya make use of a wide range of home remedies. We have included as many different remedies for each ailment as possible. The remedies we have selected primarily make use of plants and products that are easily available to you. We tell you how to order the few plants that are not easily found but that we have included because they are so effective.

Throughout we provide recipes for remedies and occasionally some culinary recipes for foods with preventive qualities. "Quick Relief," "From the Kitchen," and "Ancient Wisdom" are highlighted throughout the book as sidebars.

Part III, on bodywork, explains the philosophy behind Maya massage and outlines techniques that you can perform on yourself or a friend. You may find it odd at first that massage is included in a book about Maya home remedies, but massage is integral to the practice of Maya medicine. The Maya have a unique perspective on massage. As far as we know, nothing else has been written on the subject.

Part IV, on spiritual healing, is a must-read. You will learn about how the Maya define and treat spiritual illnesses. Here you will find rituals and prayers as well as remedies. It is our hope that you'll be rewarded with a deeper understanding of problems we all have but often don't understand.

Let us not forget the medicinal plants—the heroes and heroines of these pages. We tell you about plants that are found in the rainforest and others that you may find in your own backyard, in your spice cabinet, or at a store. We provide step-by-step directions for creating your own healing garden of medicinal plants. To help you find out more about plants that interest you, we have provided a listing of Latin names for plants at the end of the book. We have also included a list of resources that can help you locate herbs, seeds, information, and practitioners.

Whatever remedies you try, be sure to use common sense at all times. Watch for side effects, be alert for allergic reactions, be aware ahead of time of possible interactions between herbs and drugs, and always remain in touch with your physician. Stop taking the herbs immediately if you experience any adverse effects. If you are pregnant, some remedies may not be appropriate. Look in the section on women's ailments for suggestions about what you can do.

Important Spanish Healing Terms

Susto (soost-oh): fright
Pesar (pay-sar): grief
Invidia (in-vid-ee-ah): envy
Tristeza (tree-stez-ah): sadness
Bajos (bah-hose): herbal steam bath
Ciro (seer-oh): stomach complaint
Mal ojo (mal oh-ho): evil eye
Pinchar (peen-char): primitive Maya acupuncture system
Ventosa (ven-tow-sah): cupping
Viento (vee-en-toh): wind
Sobadera (sow-bah-dare-ah): Maya massage therapist
Espiritos (eh-speer-ih-tows): spirits
Hechisero (ech-ih-sayr-oh): a person who performs evil magic
Curandero (kuhr-an-dare-oh): a person who cures; a healer

Remember that self-diagnosis can be dangerous. Although bush doctors can do some amazing things under dire circumstances, there will always be a need for modern physicians. This book is *not* a first-aid manual for emergency situations. *Maya medical wisdom is an additional perspective, not a replacement for visiting your health-care provider.*

This book is written as a source of information only. The information contained in this book should by no means be considered a substitute for the advice, decisions, or judgment of the reader's physician or other professional advisor.

All efforts have been made to ensure the accuracy of the information contained in this book as of the date published. The authors and the publisher expressly disclaim responsibility for any adverse effects arising from the use or application of the information contained herein.

NOTES
1. Eric Thompson, 1930, 68–69.

PART I

Introduction to Maya Medicine

Far too many people think of the Maya as a people from the past, perhaps because of all the attention focused on the fascinating cities that their ancestors left behind. I too am thrilled at the sight of the ancient temples, palaces, and mounds scattered throughout Belize and Central America. Ix Chel Farm, my home, is built on top of one.

Having lived among the Maya for thirty years, I can assure you that they are very much alive! Many of their twenty-eight languages are still spoken today throughout parts of Mexico, Guatemala, Belize, Honduras, and El Salvador. In addition to their languages, some of their ancient traditions remain intact. Maya medicine is one of the richest traditions to have survived the destruction wrought by the Spaniards.

Maya architectural, astronomical, mathematical, and engineering feats have fascinated us for generations, but few people are aware of their sophisticated and effective medical system. When I first began working with Don Elijio in 1982, I was mainly interested in absorbing his knowledge of plants and herbal remedies so that I could incorporate it into my own healing practice. Although I had lived alongside the Maya and the Nahuatl Indians in southern Mexico for years, I knew next to nothing about their large body of medicinal knowledge.

Only gradually did it dawn on me that Don Elijio and the Maya had much more to offer than just plant knowledge. Indeed, their knowledge and use of plants is only one, albeit very important, part of their worldview.

Anthropologists consider Maya medicine a medical-religious system. In essence the Maya have a two-pronged approach to healing. They have remedies for a wide range of physical ailments that any individual or health practitioner would be pleased to add to a healing repertoire. As part of the visible world, physical ailments—like stomachaches or infected wounds—are handled with "natural-empirical" or "naturalistic" knowledge.

The Maya have equally effective remedies, however, for the ailments of the spirit that the human eye cannot see, such as sadness, grief, fright, and envy. They are part of the "magical-mystical" world, and have traditionally been the responsibility of the h'men. Maya healers believe that these ailments involving the soul and spirits are "supernatural" in origin, and that supernatural forces can both sicken and heal.

The natural and supernatural bodies of knowledge are intertwined. For example, Maya plant lore does not exist in a state of separation from the human soul. This concept is sometimes difficult for the modern mind, trained in separatist ideology from infancy, to grasp. The union of these two worlds allows Maya medicine to go beyond "modern medicine."

I am especially taken with Maya spirits, the concept of spiritual illness, and spiritual healing. I love the way the Maya spirits are an intimate part of daily life—respected in so many activities, not just during a weekly appointment in a church or synagogue. Maya spiritual healing can help fill the emptiness and longing at the root of so much illness.

Over the years I have begun to find the "magical" side of Maya medicine extremely useful—for both my patients and myself. The Maya paradigm has opened doors that I never imagined existed. Their ideas about spiritual illness have helped me understand why some people get well and some don't, even when their illnesses and treatments are the same.

There is plenty of room for this kind of wisdom in our modern culture. Since the 1960s Westerners have been storming the gates of Eastern healing traditions, and that intense interest has not subsided. We suggest that it would be wise to look south and add Maya wisdom to our banks of planetary knowledge.

Traditional healing is a tapestry that has been woven by humans throughout history. The patterns reverberate from culture to culture, and the themes are universal. Much of what you will read here about the Maya will resonate with what you know intuitively. Although the Maya contribution to the tapestry has been neglected, the colors and patterns remain, reflecting world wisdom for those who choose to see.

Every once in a great while the folly of one century becomes the common sense of the next. The time of the Maya has arrived. Time, you might say, has caught up with them. Or perhaps it is just that the rest of us have finally caught on.

There is a legend that the old godlike prophet-king of the Maya and Aztecs will return one day. He is known as Quetzalcoatl to the Aztecs and Kukulcan to the Maya. Both of these names refer to the "plumed serpent" or "feathered snake." The snake has been a symbol of medicine and healing power since ancient times for many cultures around the world, including the Maya.

This great god-king prophesied that white men would come to these lands on "the wings of a dove," and that men would lead them with two different feet. One foot would be that of a dove and the other that of an eagle. The white people would claim to be doves but would act like eagles. They would eventually steal the red man's land, religion, women, and dignity, and the ensuing period of slavery and suffering would last for hundreds of years.

Then one day other white men would appear with both feet like those of the doves, proclaiming love and brotherhood. These are the ones who would join the red man in an era of renewal, respect, and reverence for the nearly lost ancient ways. Gradually, says the prophecy, the red man will regain his former position and join the white men with the feet of doves in building a better world.

Six Principles of Maya Medicine

Here are the basic principles of Maya medicine as still practiced throughout Central America today.

1. Ch'ulel, or Life Energy

Like other indigenous cultures from Alaska to Brazil, the Maya recognize and honor the sacred within all forms of life. Plants, trees, stones, animals, and humans are all sacred.

Everything in creation is permeated with what the Maya call ch'ulel—a vibrant energy force that the Maya believe emanates from a divine spiritual source. The Maya see the entire cosmos as imbued with ch'ulel—houses, mountains, springs, sacred places, the sky, the earth.

The word *ch'ulel* has the same root as *ch'ul,* or *k'ul,* a word used by the ancient Maya to describe holiness and divinity.[1] The ancient Maya kings were called *ch'ul ahaw,* lords of the life force. *Ch'ul* is also one of the Maya words for soul.

Ch'ulel is akin to *Qi* or *chi*—the energy force described in Chinese medicine, the Indians' *prahna,* the Huna's *mana,* and the Voodoo *mojo.* Although missing from modern medicine, the concept of life force is found in healing and spiritual beliefs around the world and has been around as long as humans have been around. Look for it in cabalistic writings and traditions, the works of pre-Socratic Greeks such as Heraclitus, the teachings of the Ojibwa, and pantheism. In contemporary popular culture it is no less than "the force" in *Star Wars.* Whatever the culture, ch'ulel is a universal truth that allows us to weave our disparate selves into the fabric of the world.

If all of nature is imbued with ch'ulel, it makes sense that Maya healers can use plants, stones, animals, minerals, water, and especially prayers to heal. At the very heart of Maya medicine is the concept that medicine is all around us. We pass it daily right on our very doorstep; we also find it at roadsides and in trees, plants, stones, animals, dreams, and prayers. The Earth Mother is the great wellspring of medicinal power.

Sharing Ch'ulel with Wild Animals

In Yucatec Maya communities a *chanul* is a supernatural guardian or protector. A chanul shares ch'ulel with a person from birth and usually takes the form of a wild animal. In shamanic terminology a chanul is sometimes called a "power animal."

Belief has it that when a person is born, a corresponding chanul is born in the spirit world. This chanul remains corralled there until called forth to assist and protect. Some shamans call upon chanuls for help. Others, like Don Elijio's teacher Jeronimo Requena, have the ability to transform themselves into their chanuls. They can transfer their ch'ulel to their chanul.

Prayer also resides in the heart of the Maya system. Prayer sends the ch'ulel where it is needed, focusing it like a laser beam or energy conduit and thus leading to transformation. It is like a magnet: prayer attracts ch'ulel.

In an interview in *Omni* magazine, the late Maya scholar Linda Schele explained: "The important interactions in life are not between human and human, human and place, human and animal but between the ch'ulel and those things. Humans can lose some of their ch'ulel, then need to go through ceremonies to get it back."

The concept of soul, or ch'ulel, loss is a common shamanic theme. The Zinacanteco Maya believe that the ch'ulel has thirteen parts.[2] Illness occurs if one or more of these parts leave. Soul loss is a very important concept: many of the Maya healing traditions— including the most practical, hands-on ones—call or lure the soul back into the body. One of the main goals of Maya healing is to balance the flow of ch'ulel that moves in and out of the body.

2. No Separation of the Spiritual and Physical Realms

It follows then that if energy is everywhere, there can be no separation of mind and body and soul. Ch'ulel is present in each, and each is equally important to human health, well-being, stability, and the achievement of that elusive state of balance— human happiness.

To the Maya the spiritual and physical realms are a continuum separated only by what I imagine as a translucent gossamer veil through which the h'men has the power to penetrate. Woven throughout the veil are human emotions, which are expressed in both physical and spiritual ways.

The veil is translucent because the two realms need to be visible to each other. They need regular contact to stay in balance. There are a number of ways in which humans can peek through the veil and communicate with the spiritual realm. Among the most important are prayer, dream visions, ritual, and ceremony.

What is on the other side of the veil? The Maya cosmology is complex and based on confusing sources, so I am going to explain it as Don Elijio explained it to me. He said that the other side of the veil is where the Maya spirits live. Don Elijio loved to talk about the Maya spirits, which he called his *muy buenos amigos,* or very good friends. Indeed, he addressed these spirits as if they were his friends. He believed that they would be lonely if they were not actively involved in human affairs, and that they especially loved healing and healers.

Who are these spirits?

The spirits are manifestations of ch'ulel, and the purveyors of ch'ulel. They work alongside human beings and respond to their prayers. This is why the Maya healer believes that when a person's ch'ulel becomes depleted, prayer helps to fill it up again.

Don Elijio had special relationships with certain spirits whom I came to know through him as the Nine Benevolent Spirits. In Spanish these are known as *Los Nueve Espiritos Beneficos de los Maya* or, in Mayan, *Bolon Tiku*. Don Elijio called them *Bolon Ik*.

"They are not God, but they are the right hands of God," he used to say. "They do God's work. They are the Lords of Thunder, Lightning, Rain, Corn, and the Forest."

The Maya have a lovely image to describe the spiritual world behind the veil. In its center is a giant ceiba tree—also known as the

The Story of the Popul Vuh

The Popul Vuh is the great religious and mythological epic of the Maya. Similar to the Bible and Greek mythology, it tells the story of the creation of human beings, and in it you are sure to notice universal themes.

The Popul Vuh recounts the journeys of mythological heroes and describes the world of the Maya gods. "The myth is thought to be a compilation of many myths, and as such has a much deeper meaning than the story itself implies; it tells of the ancient Maya's ideals and beliefs and broadens our insight to ancient Mayan culture," explains James A. Fox, a Popul Vuh scholar at Stanford University.[3]

The story starts with the gods who create the earth and cover it with animals and plants. They long to create beings who will "walk, work, and talk in an articulate and measured way, visiting shrines, giving offerings, calling upon their makers by name."[4]

This is easier said than done. The divine progenitors first fashion beings from mud. When the mud beings fail to live up to expectations, the gods create a race of wooden beings. These are replaced by beings made from flesh. These first flesh beings, however, turn to wickedness. A great flood sweeps the earth and destroys them.

The gods decide to seek the counsel of an elderly god-couple named Xpiyacoc and Xmucane. According to Dennis Tedlock, Xpiyacoc is the "divine matchmaker" and Xmucane the "divine midwife." They are "daykeepers" or "diviners" who are older than other gods.

kapok tree—the denizen of the rainforest. In Mayan the tree is called *yax che*. *Yax* has three meanings: green, first, and sacred. *Che* is tree.

The trunk and branches of the tree are above the earth. The roots are below. The root level represents the underworld, and the upper world is the trunk and branches.

The branch world and root world of the tree of life mirror each other: one is dark, one is light; one is seen, one is not; one is yin, one is yang. One gathers nourishment, one is nourished. The underworld and the upper world couch our physical world. The realm in which we reside separates the two worlds and at the same time serves as the portal between them.

The ancient Maya cosmos is a trinity. One tree, three worlds. Within this trinity the Maya, like other cultures, have a dualistic

At this point the authors of the Popul Vuh turn their attention to the adventures of the heroic gods who make the sky and earth safer places for human habitation. They focus mostly on the twin sons of Xpiyacoc and Xmucane—Hunaphu (no relation to the god Hunabku) and Xbalanque, who are known as the Hero Twins.

To make a long story short, Hunaphu and Xbalanque tame the Lords of Death—the gods of the Maya underworld, which is called Xibalba.

Each time the Xibalbans try to kill them, the twins cleverly evade death. Eventually they make the Lords of Death so angry that they know they will be killed, so they arrange their own deaths in a way that allows them to be reborn. When the twins come back to life, they defeat the Lords of Death, banishing them forever from the world of humans.

Once the Hero Twins force the dark and wild forces of the universe underground, the stage is set for the fourth creation, the one in which we live today. The authors of the Popul Vuh return again to their original question—the creation of humans.

"The Gods get news of a mountain filled with yellow white corn and Xmucane—the divine midwife—grinds the corn from this mountain very finely, and the flour, mixed with the water she rinses her hands with, provides the substance for human flesh," explains Tedlock.[5]

Four men are created out of this dough. They are everything the gods want. In fact, they can see the world with as much clarity as the gods can. Feeling threatened, the gods put a "fog" on human vision and then fashion four wives for the new men. From here on the Popul Vuh tracks the history of the Quiche Maya.

view—they see the world as an eternal struggle between above and below, between good and evil.

In the upper world the trunk of the tree has thirteen levels. These are the levels of heaven where there is light and grace and goodness and forgiveness. This is a place of sunlight, growth, and regeneration. Altogether there are thirteen spirits who live above-ground. Together they are called *Oxlahuntiku* in Maya. Don Elijio called them *Oxlahunik*.

Don Elijio's beloved Nine Benevolent Spirits reside on the first nine levels. In general it is they who make daily life possible. They are the oversouls, like the archangels in the Christian tradition. They bring the rain, the thunder, and the seasons and cause all life to thrive and grow. They are the caretakers of the world who look after the people, the animals, the plants, the harvests, the seasons, the day and the night, the crossroads, women in childbirth, and all aspects of daily life. Each spirit is entrusted with certain aspects of life, and their roles often overlap in a confusing way.

The names of these spirits possess a powerful charge of ch'ulel. As a result, Don Elijio believed that their names cannot be revealed to those who do not possess a sastun. This is a real Maya secret—one of the few things I can't tell you. According to the Popul Vuh—the great spiritual text of the Maya—knowing the names of the spirits weakens their powers.

However, the names of several Maya spirits are household words among the Maya. Ix Chel, for instance, is the goddess of medicine, childbirth, weaving, and the moon, and the queen of all the goddesses. She watches over the sick, women in childbirth, newborns, the healers, and the plants. Ix Chel is the guardian of the forest, and queen of the forest spirits—what Don Elijio called the *duenos* (in Spanish, overseers or lords) or lords of the forest.

Itzamna, the male god of healing, is thought to be the consort of Ix Chel. Both he and Ix Chel wear snakes on their heads, the symbol of medicine. According to David Freidel, Linda Schele, and Joy Parker, *itz* is another Maya word for soul. *Itzam* literally means "one who does itz" or an *itzer,* another term for a shaman. They interpreted this to mean that the shaman is the person who opens the portal to bring *itz*—or soul—into the physical world.[6]

Numbers Are Sacred

Numbers are another powerful manifestation of ch'ulel. The Maya consider all the numbers between zero—which some believe the Maya invented—and thirteen to be sacred. Because there are Nine Benevolent Spirits and Nine Malevolent Spirits, nine is an especially sacred and ubiquitous number in Maya culture. Four, nine, and thirteen have the highest concentrations of ch'ulel. As you will see, these sacred numbers show up again and again in treatments in their healing system. For example, it is common to say nine prayers at one time, combine four different plants in a formula, and make a treatment out of nine different plants.

one

two

three

four

five

six

seven

eight

nine

ten

eleven

twelve

thirteen

Maya scholars have uncovered the names of other Maya spirits. For example, Yax Tum Bak is the lord of plantings, and Chac is the Maya god of rain. According to Sylvanus G. Morley, the corn god is Yum Kaax.[7]

Residing above the Nine Benevolent Spirits are the spirits who live on each of the four higher levels of heaven. At the leafy crown of the tree resides Hunabku, the ruling Spirit and the Maya's great holy God, overseeing all of creation. As Don Elijio told it, Hunabku is the father of Ix Chel and Itzamna. Hunabku and the other spirits on this level are the most powerful.

In the roots of the tree are the nine levels of the underworld, each ruled over by its own lord or spirit. These are the Nine Malevolent Spirits, who send death and destruction in the form of droughts, floods, hurricanes, war, misery, suffering, and famine.

The underworld—a central theme throughout Maya healing—is riddled with gloomy, dark passageways and tunnels. These passageways are full of suffering spirits known as "lost souls."

3. Reverence for Plants and Natural Cycles

The three worlds of the ceiba tree are connected by sap, which is the ch'ulel. Ch'ulel, constantly circulating throughout all parts of the tree, is the movement of life above and below the ground.

Thus, every plant is a sacred part of the living tapestry. All that springs from the earth is imbued with ch'ulel. As a result, all that springs from the earth has a soul. Maya healers believe that plants have *dueños*—akin to the East Indian *devas* and to Celtic elves and fairies. The Spanish word *duenos* means overseers or lords, and in modern usage it also means owner. The Mopan Maya word used by Don Elijio is *canan*. A canan is a guardian.

Plants are part of the web of healing, and their role is revered. Healing with plants has been an integral part of life on earth since the earliest times, and like other cultures, the Maya have their own vast body of plant knowledge.

Today in Maya villages great care and love are put into backyard kitchen gardens where healing plants are cultivated. The Maya understand the need to have plants close at hand and share cuttings and seeds with their neighbors.

How the Maya Re-create Creation Through Corn

In the second century B.C. the gods laid down the three stones of the cosmic hearth, which are thought to be the three stars in the constellation of Orion, according to Freidel, Schele, and Parker.[8] Even today the hearth in many traditional Maya homes is made of three stones. On it each morning the Maya woman replicates the actions of Xmucane, the mother of the Hero Twins. She builds a fire between the three stones, says a prayer, and lays a flat clay plate on top of the stones. She grinds corn, makes it into dough, and pats the dough into tortillas. She places the tortillas on the hot clay plate, where the dough balloons up to form a *panza,* or belly. The Maya see the tortilla as an analog of a human being.

The Maya man also reenacts creation while at work in his milpa. He is said to be centering the universe when he marks the four corners and sides of his cornfield.

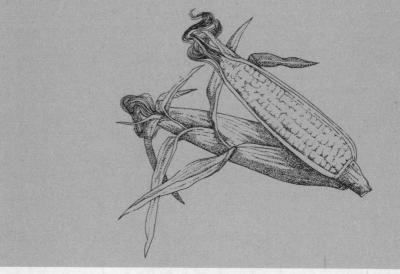

Maya healers have very personal relationships with plants. They treat them like members of the family and consider them allies in their healing work. They talk to them as if they were human friends since they believe that duenos respond, as would any living being, with their own intelligence. Don Elijio used to say about plants: "Yo les adoro, son mis muy buenos amigos" (I adore them, they are my best friends).

Healers often develop an especially strong relationship with one or two plants. Don Elijio's faithful ally was skunk root, which he relied on when all else failed. It was revealed to me in a dream that my personal plant ally is rue. I consider rue my spiritual safety net and call upon it if all else fails.

For the Maya, corn, or maize, is the most sacred and revered of all plants. Corn is considered the giver of life and the food of the gods. As is written in the Popul Vuh, the Maya believe that they themselves were created from corn.

Corn is both medicine and the symbol of rebirth. As Don Elijio taught me, the farmer buries the seed in the earth of his *milpa*—his plot of land for farming. It then dies and goes into the underworld. After Chac, the rain god, comes and prepares the earth, the corn is reborn into the upper world.

When Don Elijio was young, the entire community participated in corn ceremonies called *primicias*. These were held to

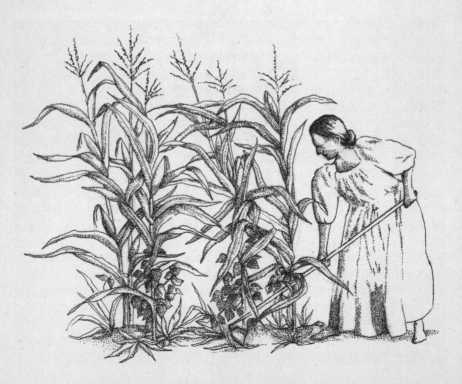

The Sap of the World

There is a Maya belief that certain times of the day or month are most felicitous for the harvesting of medicinal plants. This concept, based on the flow of ch'ulel in plants, is a wonderful example of the basic connection between the spiritual and physical worlds.

Traditional herbal practitioners feel that the night draws the healing power of a plant down into the roots and that the sun draws it up into the stems, leaves, and flowers. Therefore it is best to wait to collect leaves until the sun has risen in the sky and warmed the day. Additionally, since the watery dew can dilute some of the essential oils that make many herbs effective, allowing the dew to dry on the leaf before it is picked ensures that the oils are at their highest potency.

The phase of the moon is also believed to affect the flow of sap in plants. Central American farmers and gardeners can often be heard to comment: "It is not the right moon for planting pumpkins, corns, or beans until next week when the moon changes."

We could dismiss these beliefs as folklore, but there is scientific evidence to support their validity. Experiments have shown that water moves up in plants during the day and downward at night. The effects of the moon on fluids are well known. Not only do the tides rise and fall with the moon, but childbirth, menstruation, and human behavior are also affected.

In the rainforest a builder cutting hardwood logs for house construction works during the full-moon phase—three days before and three days after the full moon. This schedule ensures that the bitter toxic sap of the hardwood remains in the trunk so that after the tree is felled the sap will serve to deter insect infestation.

thank plants for their generosity, love, and healing power. Primicias were also held to ask for rain. During his lifetime Don Elijio regularly conducted primicias, but they ceased being community events.

4. Healing as a Team Process

The Maya view healing as a process that occurs when the spirits, plants, healer, and patient work together in good faith. No true healing occurs unless the spirits and plants are included and revered through prayer.

The Wind Is Divine

In a land of changing winds and pervading dampness, the Maya are rightfully concerned about the harmful effects of winds. They think of winds as powerful manifestations of ch'ulel. The word for wind in Mayan is *ik,* which is the same word for breath and spirit.

Like spirits, some winds are malevolent while others are benevolent. The Maya think it best to avoid the night wind at all cost. Even on an unbearably hot night Don Elijio would insist on fastening all the wooden shutters over the windows of his thatched roof hut to keep out the meandering wind spirits of the night.

Many times Don Elijio said: "People watch me prepare medicine and then go home and try to do what they saw me do. They come back and say, 'I did it as you did, and it didn't work,' and I answer them, 'Ahhh, you didn't say the prayers.'"

Much of healing boils down to faith. In a system like the Maya's, healing does not occur without faith. Let's imagine ch'ulel as a passenger in a car. If prayer is the "driver" of ch'ulel, faith is the vehicle. In other words, the healer and the patient must believe and express their faith through meaningful prayer, ritual, and ceremony.

Most traditional treatments involve prayers said by the practitioner for the patient. Some patients have said that when they receive healing prayers they experience a physical sensation of tremendous energy, a force they describe as a strong, pushing wind passing through their body. Such is ch'ulel.

5. "Asking the Blood"

For as long as the science of medicine has been around, the blood has fascinated physicians. The science of the blood is called humoral medicine, and it is practiced by at least three major traditions—Hippocrates and the Graeco-Persian-Arab, the Ayurvedic of India, and the Chinese.[9]

The Maya believe that the blood contains ch'ulel, and they use the blood for both the treatment and diagnosis of physical and spiritual problems.

How do healers use the blood for diagnosis? Traditional Maya healers are known as "pulse doctors" because the first step of their basic clinical procedure is to listen to and feel the pulse. The Kekchi Maya of southern Belize call this "asking the blood."[10] The Zinacanteco Maya, who live near San Cristobal de las Casas in the Chiapas Mountains in Mexico, say that the blood "speaks" to the healer. "The blood 'speaks' to the h'ilol [seer, another word for healer], who knows how to pulse, and reveals the nature of the illness and the cure that is demanded," according to Daniel Silver.[11]

Within only a few moments, a practiced healer can determine a great deal of information about a patient from the pulse. Don Elijio once listened to a woman's pulse and knew correctly that she had had surgery three months earlier. He could also determine whether a health problem was of spiritual or physical origin.

The pulse diagnosis determines the treatment the healer chooses. Before the healer does anything else, he or she always says nine prayers into the pulse to help recharge and rebalance the flow of ch'ulel in and out of the body. This is a wonderful tradition that transfers energy from spirits to healer to patient. "The great chain of transmission leads back to God," said James Boster.[12]

This helps explain the ancient Maya's devotion to bloodletting. Ancient healers believed that bloodletting releases any negative ch'ulel that may have accumulated. It also releases positive ch'ulel to the gods. Bloodletting was especially popular among the royalty, who were thought to have the most powerful life force—the strongest concentrations of ch'ulel. When Maya kings pierced their tongues and penises, they believed that they were feeding the gods their ch'ulel and giving of their souls.

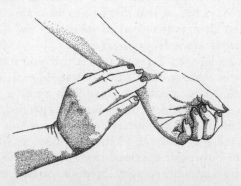

6. The Theory of Hot and Cold

The concept of hot and cold underlies just about every remedy of the Maya, even their bodywork. As you will see, "hot" and "cold" do not refer only to temperature.

The ch'ulel in the blood is affected by hot and cold. When the ch'ulel is hot, it speeds the pulse and causes ailments whose symptoms include fever and swelling. When the ch'ulel is cold, it slows the pulse, causing ailments that feature stiffness and chills.

When the Maya use the word "cold" in a therapeutic setting, they mean closed and congested. When the Maya use the word "hot," they mean open and flowing.

Ailments are either cold or hot. Cold ailments exhibit chills, cramping, paralysis, or constipation. Hot ailments exhibit fever, diarrhea, vomiting, and boils.

Ailments are treated with hot or cold remedies. The Maya believe that foods and plants are either hot or cold. Some hot foods are chocolate, garlic, onions, peppers, coffee, and ginger. Cheese, which thickens mucus, is considered a cold food.

Some hot plants are rue, rosemary, and coffee. Desert nopal, roses, and mallows are among the cold plants. Nopal, a cold plant, is used to treat sunburn, while ginger, a hot plant, is given for stomach cramps, which is considered a cold condition. Hot remedies often counteract the symptoms of ailments that occur in the cooler weather, while cold remedies counteract the effects of hot weather.

A key belief in Central America and the Caribbean is that a quick change in temperature is the root cause of many physical ailments. The Maya believe that it is best to maintain equilibrium and avoid sudden changes that lead to what they call "blood shock," also called *vientos* (winds) or *aires* (airs).

A Maya healer would never suggest that you jump into a cold pool once you have worked up a sweat. Nor would he or she approve of drinking a cold beverage with a hot meal. The Maya reasoning is that the sudden cold causes the expanded, warm muscles to spasm, thereby causing illness.

Scholars are still debating whether the concept of hot and cold originated in Europe or developed on its own in the New World. Some of the sixteenth-century Spanish priests who translated

Mesoamerican medical texts mentioned the Maya fascination with hot and cold. However, it is unclear whether their Old World concepts influenced their translations.[13]

The Story of Maya Healing

Modern scholars have been studying the Maya ever since the ancient Maya cities were brought to popular attention in 1841 through the writings of John L. Stephens and the illustrations of Frederick Catherwood. The publication of *Incidents of Travel in Central America, Chiapas, and Yucatan* was the beginning of a love affair with the Maya that has never let up.

We know now that the forebears of the Maya and other indigenous Mesoamericans (and for that matter the human populations of the New World) crossed the Bering Strait at the end of the Pleistocene Ice Age. By 7000 B.C. the ice sheets had melted and the climate began to warm up. Corn may have come under cultivation around 5000 B.C.[14]

Near Veracruz, Mexico, Olmec civilization emerged around 1200–900 B.C. The Olmec are considered the "mother" of Mesoamerican civilizations. Maya villages are thought to have begun forming around 1000 B.C. The population grew, spreading to what is now Belize, Guatemala, western parts of Honduras and El Salvador, and the Yucatan, Tabasco, and Chiapas in Mexico. The Maya began to build cities and to distinguish themselves in writing, art, astronomy, engineering, and architecture.

"During a span of six centuries, from about A.D. 300 to 900, the Maya, particularly those of the Central area, reached intellectual and artistic heights which no others in the New World, and few in the Old, could match at that time," said Michael Coe. "The Classic period was a kind of Golden Age, not only for them but for the rest of the Mesoamerican peoples."[15]

The great Maya cities were abandoned between A.D. 900 and 980. This is a subject of much speculation among scholars. There are many hypotheses about the Maya urban demise—war, civil discontent, famine—but all we know for sure is that the Maya people ceased to maintain their sprawling cities. They left behind their grand temples, which were soon swallowed up by the rainforest to stand untouched for centuries, appearing to be no more than large hills rising mysteriously from valleys and foothills.

Over the next five hundred years the Maya passed their traditions on from generation to generation until in 1519 ominous sails appeared on the horizon. Cortez arrived on the shores of Mexico, dramatically transforming their world. The Spaniards sent troops throughout Mesoamerica to conquer the Maya and others with guns and, even more effectively, disease. Hundreds of thousands of Mesoamericans died of the diseases the Spaniards brought to the New World, especially smallpox and syphilis. These were illnesses for which their medical system had no cure and their immune systems no defense.

Along with soldiers came priests, who took it as their spiritual duty to extinguish what they considered heathen and to replace the indigenous heritage with their own. The priests fanned out through Mesoamerica, Christianizing the indigenous peoples and convincing them to accept Spanish medical practices.

Bishop Diego de Landa is infamous for his zealous destruction of Maya texts and idols. He himself is thought to have been responsible for the burning of one hundred thousand Mesoamerican texts. Another priest—Friar Juan de Zumarraga—is

Surviving Maya Writings

Only in the last decade have scholars dedicated to the study of Maya hieroglyphs, like Linda Schele, begun to understand the Maya written language. Ancient Maya leaders recorded much information about themselves on the upright carved stone slabs known as stelae. Stelae have been found at Maya archaeological sites throughout Central America.

Few books survived the Spanish Inquisition, not to mention the humid climate. In addition to the Popul Vuh there is a Quiche Maya history called *The Annals of Kaqchikel* and a play called *RabinAl Achi*. There is also *Ritual of the Bakabs,* a Yucatec Maya book of incantations. The Yucatec Maya have the books of Chilam Balam.

There are also four Maya books that came to be called *The Dresden, The Paris, The Madrid,* and *The Grolier Codices.* These were accordion-like texts made of beaten bark paper from the fig or amati tree and covered with a thin layer of plaster. They appear to be almanacs for the timing of rituals.[16]

thought to have destroyed another seven hundred thousand texts he found in Mexico.

Although much was destroyed, the Maya did resist the complete absorption of their culture and religion. They held on to their beloved spirits, traditions, gods, and goddesses by transferring their qualities to Catholic saints, thus preserving the core of their beliefs. Some Maya communities managed to remain outside Spanish influence, especially in Belize, where there were no reports of gold.

Since their healing tradition was passed down through oral tradition, the Maya held on to much of it, incorporating some Moorish and Spanish ideas. Clearly, contemporary Maya healers throughout Mesoamerica blend Old and New World beliefs. Don Elijio's religion was a happy mix of ancient Maya beliefs and Catholicism. As a healer he often called upon the Nine Benevolent Spirits and the four virgins—Carmen, Guadalupe, Fatima, and Lourdes—who when combined reflect the four aspects of the goddess of healing, Ix Chel.

Don Elijio would gaze into his sastun—the stone he used to communicate with the Maya spirits—until he found "the Virgin." He would jump up with glee and exclaim, "There she is! There she is! I see her! The Virgin Mary is there, right there!" He loved both the queen of the Christian heaven and the queen of the Maya upper world, Ix Chel. They were all like his girlfriends.

"Jesus, Mary, and saints like Michael and Gabriel came to this land of my people many centuries ago," Don Elijio once explained to me. "When they came, the Nine Maya Spirits called a heavenly council with them. They are not like you and me, you know. They are not jealous or full of envy. No, they all got together at this big meeting and decided to work together for the salvation of the people's souls. Together they answer our prayers, heal the sick, and hold our hands when we die. We pray to them, and they answer with miracles. Faith is what moves them to work for us."

Fortunately, some early Spaniards made an effort to record and preserve the Maya culture. Even Bishop Diego de Landa wrote a useful, if biased, chronicle of Maya life around 1566.

Interestingly enough, some Maya healing concepts made their way back to the Old World. In fact, early Spanish chroniclers were astounded at the sophisticated botanical gardens and research in medicinal plants conducted in the New World before Columbus was born. According to Gordon Schendel, about two thousand plants were in imperial botanical gardens in Mexico City when Cortez arrived. The botanical garden was thought to be the largest in the world at the time. The Spanish crown commanded Spanish doctors to study indigenous uses of plants and to report back with anything useful. A market developed in Europe for the Old World plants such as sarsaparilla, otherwise known as China root. "A new [medical] concept evolved, that was neither indigenous or Spanish," said Schendel. "It was unique in that each group accepted knowledge from the other."[17]

As part of his research mission, one open-minded sixteenth century Spanish priest translated the medical teachings of an indigenous healer. Several years ago, while attending an herbal conference on the East Coast of the United States, a pharmacist came up to me after my lecture and presented me with a most wonderful gift. "Here," he said, "I've had this book for many years, and when I saw your name on the roster of speakers, I decided that you should have it."

The Maya, Pagans, and Early Jews

There are powerful similarities between the Maya and pre-Judeo-Christian pagans and early Jewish beliefs (both of which heavily influenced Christianity). Pagans, like the Maya, worshiped many spirits and gods, including a god of fertility of plants, humans, and animals. Jews have a tree of life in the Garden of Eden, while the Maya have the Ceiba tree. Jews also used amulets to protect them from evil. Even today some religious Jews use "phylacteries." Early Jews believed in a wide variety of spirit-like angels, including seven archangels. "God created countless helper angels who rule the winds, the coming of day and night, and all of nature," said Miriam Chaiken.[18] When Jews began to pray to angels as if they were god, rabbis discouraged—but never fully eliminated—the belief in angels.

In his hands he held a copy of the *Badianus Manuscript*, a fascinating text prepared in 1552 and believed to be the only such manuscript in existence that does not reflect the influence of European medical practices. It is the earliest known book on the subject of healing with medicinal plants in the New World. It was found on a dusty shelf in 1929 when a monk decided to clean out an old section of the Vatican Library.

It is the work of a young Aztec Indian healer, Martinus de la Cruz, a healer of the time, and Juan Badianus, a Spanish monk who translated the text from Aztec into Latin. The book is a delightful work containing simple drawings of the medicinal plants in brilliant colors and information about treatments, prayers, and the ailments that the plants treat. Many of the diseases discussed in this text have not been identified by modern medicine.

It is generally believed that the Mesoamerican civilizations are related. Thus, the healing traditions in the *Badianus Manuscript*, though not specifically Maya, are nevertheless extremely valuable to our understanding of traditional practices.

There are more modern sources of information about the Maya healing traditions. Ralph Roys's *Ethnobotany of the Maya* was written in 1931. The sophisticated medical system of the Maya people, though always a mystery to Roys, elicited his respect and reverence. He wrote his book in both Mayan and English, and it is an excellent source of Mayan names for medicinal plants and their uses. Roys tells of the changes that took place in Maya medicine as a result of the Spanish conquest. For instance, he traces the origins of an ancient medical practice called *ventosa*, or cupping, to Spain, then to Arabia, and finally to China.

The Asian Exchange

It is important to note that even before Europeans set foot in Mesoamerica the Maya may have exchanged ideas with early traders from the Pacific Islands. There are remarkable similarities between Maya and Asian ideas about medicine, some of which can be attributed to the Asian origin of the Maya people. It is also possible that myths, rituals, and concepts from India and China traveled to the islands of the Pacific, and from there to Mesoamerica.

The latest blow to the Maya medical tradition was the double punch of evangelism and the ascent of modern medicine, which together came close to destroying the oral healing tradition. Protestant evangelism, which began to sweep through Central America in the 1950s and continues to this day, is intolerant of the Maya religion. The evangelists are bent on cleaning up old

Catholicism and have replaced all gods and goddesses with Jesus. Their intolerance extends to the Maya's traditional medical system.

Fortunately, other factors have led to a resurgence of interest in Maya medicine, among both the Maya themselves and the rest of the world. Modern medicine has begun to open its doors to the possibility that there is more to healing than laboratory chemistry. At the same time modern culture has become more respectful of indigenous cultures. Average Maya have begun to take pride—once again—in their healing heritage. One manifestation of this has been the establishment of traditional healers' associations.

About ten years ago healers in Belize founded the Traditional Healers Foundation (THF). Another group is the Association of Traditional Healers of Chiapas, in the Tzotzil Maya region around San Cristobal de las Casas in Mexico. Groups like these work to keep the religious and medical traditions of the Maya alive and are opening centers to provide care and training. They are also fighting for a share of the profits from drugs that have been developed from local plants, based on traditional knowledge.

The plants of the rainforest have also been garnering more respect. For decades they have been succumbing to development and traditional slash-and-burn agriculture. Since the 1970s the World Health Organization (WHO), the United Nations Education, Scientific, and Cultural Organization (UNESCO), and other international groups have been emphasizing the importance of gathering information about medicinal plants before they disappear.

In the 1980s the U.S. National Cancer Institute contracted with the Missouri Botanical Garden in St. Louis, the University of Illinois in Chicago, and the New York Botanical Garden to gather thousands of plants in the world's rainforests. Extracts from leaves, flowers, barks, and roots were screened for anticancer and anti-AIDS properties.

We at the Ix Chel Tropical Research Foundation—under the direction of Dr. Michael Balick, director of the Institute of Economic Botany and associate vice president for research and training at the New York Botanical Garden—traveled throughout the bush to collect thousands of plant specimens. As part of our project we interviewed traditional healers from various cultural backgrounds in Belize.

We were not the only ones searching for possible cures for human ailments in Central America. Another group is led by Dr. Brent Berlin and his wife, Elois, anthropologists at the University of Georgia's Center for Latin America and Caribbean Studies. They have spent more than a decade collecting information about how the highland Maya in Chiapas use various plants to treat a wide range of illnesses. A recent study conducted by the Berlins highlights the impressive abilities and plant knowledge of Maya traditional healers.

The Traditional Healers Foundation and the Terra Nova Medicinal Plant Reserve

In the late 1980s the Ix Chel Tropical Research Foundation organized several traditional healers' conferences funded by the agency U.S. Aid for International Development (USAID). There were five conferences in all—the first of their kind ever to take place in Belize.

Hundreds of traditional healers and members of the public came to the conferences. One workshop was about the problems and concerns of traditional healers. A major concern was the rapid disappearance of the rainforest due to destruction for agriculture, development, and community expansion. The rainforest is the healers' storehouse of medicinal plants. Without it they cannot practice their art. "It would be like a mechanic without tools," explained the midwife Hortence Robinson.

Everyone agreed that we needed to establish an organization to promote traditional healing, encourage apprentices to follow in the old ways, and represent the interests of traditional healers at the government level. Thus the Traditional Healers Foundation was formed. The THF was also mandated to look after the intellectual property rights of the healers who participate in scientific and pharmaceutical research programs.

The foundation's first project was to petition the government of Belize for a tract of rainforest land to be set aside for the express purpose of conserving medicinal plants and preserving traditional healing. The minister of natural resources, the Honorable Daniel Silva, loved the idea and identified a tract of old-growth rainforest in the Yalbac region of Cayo District in western Belize.

When we looked at the map and did a preliminary walkabout in the area, it was clear that the six-thousand-acre site was perfect. The reserve, funded by grants from all over the world, is known as the Terra Nova (New Earth) Forest Reserve.

"Our data shows that the Highland Maya have developed a large number of herbal remedies based on astute understanding of the signs and symptoms of common disease condition," the Berlins wrote recently. "Furthermore, the potential therapeutic efficacy of Maya herbal medicine is suggested by laboratory studies on the pharmacological properties affecting the agents associated with the ethnomedically identified clinical signs and symptoms that correlate closely with bio-molecular medical disease categories."[19]

While the plant knowledge of the Maya gains more respect, interest in Maya spiritual healing practices has grown as well. One part of that healing practice—shamanism—has received quite a bit of attention. A number of contemporary researchers have been studying Maya shamans throughout Mesoamerica. In 1993 David Freidel, Linda Schele, and Joy Parker wrote *Maya Cosmos: Three Thousand Years on the Shaman's Path,* about a shaman named Don Pablo in Yaxuba in the Yucatan. Barbara Tedlock is another well-respected scholar who has studied shamanism. Both she and the Maya scholar Duncan Earle have become shamans themselves. Many Central American shamans are now the subjects of popular books and university treatises.

This new burst of interest is wonderful, but until now few have addressed the full complexity of the Maya's comprehensive healing system. In this book we hope to weave together the many threads of Maya medicine in an effort to keep this tradition from vanishing from this earth anytime soon.

Maya Traditional Healers in Belize

Another name for the *h'men,* the "one who knows," is *itzer,* which means "doer." The Kekchi Maya use the word *h'ilonel,* which means seer. The Tzutujil Maya call their master curer *ajkun.*[20]

Whatever the title, the h'men is the doctor-priest or priestess who has the experience, power, and mandate to deal with both physical and spiritual ailments. He or she can contact the spirit world on the other side of the veil to ask for assistance in the diagnosis and treatment of ailments.

The h'men is similar to what we commonly call a shaman. The word *shaman* comes from the Tungus people of Siberia and usually refers to a witch, witch doctor, medicine man, sorcerer, wizard, magician, or seer, explains the shamanic expert Michael Harner. "Shamans—whom we in the 'civilized' world have called 'medicine men' and 'witch doctors'—are the keepers of a remarkable body of ancient techniques that they use to achieve and maintain well-being and healing for themselves and members of their communities," writes Harner.[21]

The renowned scholar Mircea Eliade observed that the shaman is distinguished by a state of consciousness that he called "ecstasy," which he defined as being able to leave the body at will.[22] While in this trancelike state the shaman's soul is believed to leave his or her body and go to the spirit world in the sky or the underworld. Interestingly enough, the Zinacanteco Maya considered epileptics prime shaman material, since epilepsy was thought to be caused by ch'ulel leaving the body to attend to the divine.[23]

It is one of the functions of the h'men to retrieve the souls of the living from the underworld. "When parts of a soul split off and vanish into non-ordinary reality, leaving a person in a weakened, dispirited condition, it is the job of the shaman to restore wholeness," explained Sandra Ingerman.[24]

Each h'men chooses his or her own healing tools. Some h'mens rely more on healing plants while others prefer shamanic journeying. Some are diviners while others are not. Whatever tools he or she uses, a h'men is always the messenger to the spirit world.

The *village healer* is a man or woman who over the years has become the health-care provider for the entire village. Often the village healer performs spiritual as well as physical healing. He or she refers the toughest cases to a h'men.

The *granny healer* is usually a woman who has raised a brood of children using only home remedies to treat common ailments. Granny healers are experienced but tend to care only for their immediate families. If unable to treat a certain condition, they rely on the help of the village healer for additional expertise.

The *midwife*, known also as a *traditional home birth attendant*, is often trained by a parent or grandparent to deliver babies in rural areas. The midwife is most often a woman, but among the Kekchi

Maya in southern Belize the husband traditionally attends the birth of his children, and young boys are trained by their fathers for this task from early childhood. Midwives are experts at dealing with the ailments of women and children and provide excellent pre- and postnatal care. After the delivery of a baby the midwife stays at or visits the home of the new mother for nine days to ensure that both mother and child are doing well (thus the term "mid-wife").

The *massage therapist,* known as the *sobadera,* can be a man or woman and is an expert at treating muscle spasms, backaches, sprains, overworked muscles, and general aches and pains. This knowledge is handed down from parent to child and is often considered a divine gift. The sobadera is much sought after in Maya communities and is considered a vital part of the fabric of society.

The *bone setter,* or *folk chiropractor,* has been trained, usually by a parent, to treat fractures, broken bones, and pulled ligaments. These healers get excellent results using ancient manipulation techniques.

The *snake doctor* treats toxic and venomous bites and stings caused by snakes, spiders, scorpions, worms, bats, rats, rabid dogs, and puncture wounds from rusty implements. This man or woman plays an essential role in the village and is trained to act as quickly as any emergency room physician would. Many snake doctors receive their patients from hospital wards where the right medication is unavailable or the patient's case has been given up as hopeless. The snake doctor's practice and formulas are secret and are usually passed on to only one person, often a family member, in a lifetime.

Pincheros practice a very primitive form of acupuncture known as *pinchar.* They use stingray spines, porcupine quills, and tree thorns rather than needles. Some eighty different points have been identified in Maya acupuncture for treating all types of diseases.

Ensalmeros, or *prayer-makers,* are people who use only prayers in their traditional healing practice. Most often found in isolated villages, ensalmeros are usually people of great faith and simplicity.

Their prayers, addressed to the usual combination of Maya gods and Christian saints, are said into the patient's pulse. These prayers are especially important in the treatment of infants and children but can help anyone.

Diviners use a variety of methods to look into the future, including throwing down corn kernels and beans. Divining is a disappearing art: h'mens are now usually responsible for divination.

Basic Tools of Maya Healing

The Maya view of the human condition is broad. A Maya healer would never expect someone to recover simply by talking out a problem, changing his or her behavior or environment, or taking a medication. Although they do use these tools (their medications are in the form of plants), their "medicine chest" has more to offer: prayer first and foremost, the sastun, medicinal plants, herbal baths, incense, holy water, dream visions, ritual and ceremony, and amulets.

In this book you will learn how to use many of these tools and techniques. Some are appropriate for home care, and some are not. You are likely to find that you have a knack for some techniques and cannot master others. Each healer chooses the tools that work for him or her. Few healers master every tool, and such mastery is not necessary for effective healing.

Prayer

Whenever I ask a Maya healer of any age, "What is your most important healing tool?" they always answer with a single word: "Prayer." Prayer (in Spanish, *ensalmo*) is at the heart of the Maya medical-religious system and is used by all traditional healers, whether snake doctor or midwife. It is the prayer that carries the ch'ulel between the physical and spiritual worlds.

Prayers are intrinsically powerful verbal sounds that embody the power of God. To recite that power is to know it. A power residing within each individual, prayer is tapped through meditation and ritual. Prayer unites the individual with the universal, the physical with the divine, and allows us to both give and receive love.

Maya prayers are very similar to the medicine songs of North American indigenous peoples: they are chants repeated nine times in a soft whisper. Some Maya prayers have been learned through dream visions, and others have been handed down from ancestors. Don Elijio taught me dozens of prayers from his memory bank, and since then I have learned more from other healers. Some prayers can be passed only from h'men to h'men and are treasured as much as the sastun.

The prayers are always repeated nine times. Three prayers are said while holding the patient's right radial pulse at the wrist, then three at the left radial pulse, and finally three more while placing both hands over the top of the skull and forehead, which the Maya believe to be the fountain of the spirit.

Prayers for infants and children are said differently. The healer makes a cross pattern over the child's body while repeating the prayer nine times. Two prayers are said while holding the pulse of

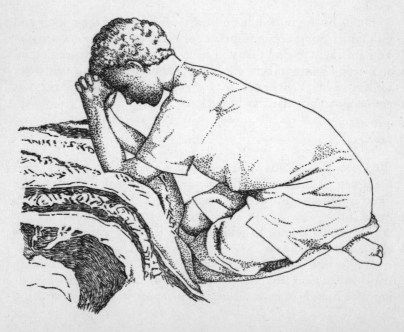

the right wrist; two over the left ankle; two over the pulse at the left wrist; two over the right ankle; and finally one last prayer is said while holding both hands over the forehead.

Prayers must be said with faith. Faith is the foundation on which all else is built in Maya medicine. This shouldn't be big news. Study after study has shown that there is a relationship between faith and the immune system. As Don Elijio used to say, "I am the one who collects and prepares the medicine, but it is faith that cures."

Soul Retrieval and Shamanic Journeying

The healer performs shamanic journeying by separating his or her ch'ulel from the body and traveling into the spirit world. There he or she seeks an answer to a problem and brings back lost ch'ulel to heal a patient. It is very common for h'mens to speak of traveling to the Maya underworld to retrieve a soul that has been lost from its body.

The concept of soul retrieval through shamanic journeying is a universal theme. Don Elijio did not practice shamanic journeying: he did not leave his body to retrieve lost souls. He accomplished soul retrieval though dreams, prayers, and the use of sacred objects such as copal incense and the sastun.

Medicinal Plants

The Maya word for medicinal plant is *xiv* (sheev). Xiv is either primary medicine in the form of vines, roots, or barks or secondary medicine from leaves and flowers.

Thousands of medicinal plants are available to the Maya healer, but each healer settles on perhaps only two dozen that he or she uses daily. Healers may use others as the need arises. The choice of plants depends on the kind of ailments being treated. For example, healers who treat spiritual ailments often collect rue, basil, marigold, and other plants known for their spiritual value, while midwives gather plants for women and children.

Plants are collected with respect, reverence, and prayer. Like all of earth's resources, plants are imbued with ch'ulel, which must be engaged so that the plant acts with full potency. "When you say the

What Is a Medicinal Plant?

Medicinal plants are defined as plants that produce one or more active ingredients capable of preventing or curing an illness. Medicinal plants contain numerous chemical compounds, which are called secondary metabolites. These are natural chemicals that the plant does not need to support its own existence, explains Margarita Artschwager Kay. "Some may be allochemicals, that is, compounds that affect other organisms in the environment and may also evoke a physiological response in humans. The concentration of metabolites depends on the part of the plant, the season of the year, and the chemistry of the soil where the plant grows." According to Kay, "this may explain why some herbalists maintain that there are certain times of years and specific places that are optimal for collecting medicinal plants."[25]

Often toxic compounds, metabolites are medicinal if used in appropriate doses; all have some effect on humans. The names of the classes of metabolites may sound familiar: alkaloids, antibiotics, glycosides, flavenoids, coumarins, tannins, bitter compounds, saponins, terpenes and essential oils, citric and tartaric acids, and mucilages.

prayer of thanksgiving and faith to the plant, the plant spirit follows you home to help with the healing," Don Elijio used to say. Without a prayer, the spiritual essence of the plant returns to the earth, and the healing is, at best, random chance.

It is also important to have faith in the plant's healing propensities. "When you go out to gather medicinal plants for your patients, don't say, 'I hope this will work,' or, 'Maybe this will work.' Clearly state your faith that it will work," Don Elijio often told me.

Medicinal plants can be prepared as teas, made into tinctures in alcohol, steeped in oil to produce a healing salve for the skin, dried and powdered for wounds, boiled with sugar to make syrups, mashed with salt to make poultices, and administered as herbal baths. Medicinal plants can also be dried, powdered, and rolled into cornhusks and smoked.

Pulses

Every Maya healer begins by checking the patient's pulse. The conduit of the body's ch'ulel, the pulsing blood provides information about the physical and spiritual condition of the patient.

The Maya go far beyond the modern medical system's use of the pulse. Medical doctors count the number of pulse beats per minute, but Maya healers recognize eighteen different kinds of pulses. They listen for strength, depth, rapidity, rhythm, location, and bounce. Only with years of practice can a healer learn the skill of recognizing the eighteen pulses. After fifteen years of integrating Maya medicine into my practice, I am still learning to differentiate the pulses.

The traditions of pulse diagnosis among the Chinese and the Maya are strikingly similar. In both practices the study of the pulse is of great importance. The Chinese consider the superficial, middle, and deep pulse, as do the Maya. The Maya take pulse diagnosis one step further, however, by using it for treatment: the healer says prayers directly into the pulse at the wrist and ankle.

When I study the Chinese theory of pulse diagnosis, it feels like I am having a chat with Don Elijio. I can see him, in his humble clinic, sitting on his little wooden stool, pointing to a patient's pulse, and tapping out the beat with his foot to teach me to listen.

Herbal Baths

If the lost art of therapeutic herbal bathing were to be rediscovered, a most useful tool would be restored to healers and physicians. Hydrotherapy—taking of the waters—and seawater therapy have been a part of the fabric of medicine since earliest times. The Maya consider water ch'ulel. It is an elixir that refreshes and purifies the body.

Herbal baths combine the power of water with that of plants. Together they absorb our pain, fear, and anxiety and leave us cleansed and renewed at a deep, energetic level. When plants are collected and prepared with prayer and loving intent, an additional energy charge is transmitted to the patient.

The Maya healer treats nearly all patients with a series of three, four, or nine herbal baths, depending on the nature of the ailment.

The Maya also use steam baths, known as *bajos*. The vaginal steam bath (pages 92–93) is a popular remedy for women's ailments.

Massage

Maya massage is one of the most useful techniques that I learned from Don Elijio. Nearly all Maya healers incorporate therapeutic touch and massage into their treatment of both spiritual and physical ailments. The sobaderas specialize in bodywork. Midwives incorporate massage into all phases of their care of women and infants. Bone setters rely heavily on a unique style of impressively deep, even painful, massage to set dislocations and heal injured ligaments.

Maya abdominal massage is the most unique aspect of Maya bodywork. It is highly effective for stomach complaints, women's ailments, and prostate problems. Don Elijio's technique of centering the uterus is an important addition to our understanding of women's health care.

Counseling

Many an unhappy person would slink into Don Elijio's clinic after dark just to talk in Maya and ask for guidance or relate a sad tale. Who can live without someone to talk to in times of need? The healers I know have become intuitive experts at compassionate listening and giving good, commonsense advice. An encouraging word, a sympathetic ear, a shared story, and a pat on the back can mean so much. A loving word is to the afflicted what sun and rain are to the earth.

Humor

Don Elijio was the funniest man I ever met. He always humbly referred to himself as "the clown of San Antonio." He could turn sad hearts around with his jokes and stories. In fact, his stories were medicine. Many other healers use humor, including some well-known American healers—like my friend and colleague Patch Adams, who was recently featured in a Hollywood movie. Humor is the best tool a healer can have in his or her bag. As Don Elijio always said: "Most people think too much, but get them to laugh and half their trouble and sickness will go away."

Ventosa

Just a few months ago my back went out and I was confined to bed. My gardener, Bernadino—a massage therapist from Don Elijio's village of San Antonio—performed ventosa on my back with a kitchen glass. It really helped.

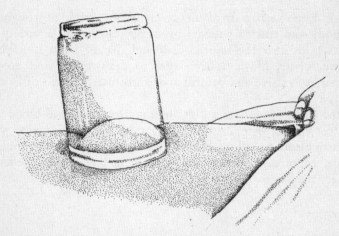

Viento in Spanish means wind, and *ventosa* means pulling out the wind. Wind, or viento, is another name for muscle spasm and tissue congestion.

Ventosa uses a combination of heat and suction to ease pain and heal congestion that comes with sciatic nerve pain, low back pain, shoulder stiffness, and injuries from falls. First, the healer lubricates the affected areas with oil. Then he or she takes a plain thick drinking glass. Beeswax or something sticky like chewing gum is used to glue a small piece of cotton to the inside surface of the glass. The cotton is set aflame and the glass turned upside down over the painful area. The glass is placed right on the skin and then moved over the affected area, pulling the flesh upward, loosening the congestion.

Similar to Chinese techniques known as cupping, ventosa is not an original Maya tradition. However, Maya healers have used this technique for hundreds of years. Ventosa is an effective technique that requires specific training and expertise.

Pinchar

Pinchar is a very primitive form of acupuncture. I have seen modern Maya healers use pinchar with stingray spines, porcupine quills, and tree thorns to relieve pain and inflammation by puncturing one or more of about eighty possible energy points on the body.

Don Elijio was aware of energy meridians running throughout the body and treated patients by using pinchar on a variety of points both near the injured area and distant from it. Unlike acupuncturists, Maya healers want to draw blood and do so. Pinchar is invasive and painful and is not used much in this day and age.

One effect of pinchar is bloodletting to release "bad blood" or negative ch'ulel. The Tzutujil Maya made small punctures with obsidian blades to "allow the bad blood to flow out," according to the anthropologist Bill Gray Douglas. "The bad blood is believed to carry the illness."[26]

Sastun

The Mayan word *sas* means light, pure, unblemished, and mirror. *Tun* means stone or age. Together they form the word *sastun* (sastoon), which can mean light of the ages, stone of the ages, and stone of light—all names for this cherished tool of divination and spiritual power. Sastun can also be spelled *zaztun* or *sastoon*.

Only Maya h'mens have a sastun, and not all of them possess one. The sastun has a super dose of ch'ulel and can be used to communicate directly with the Maya spirits. The sastun helps to diagnosis spiritual diseases.

Spirit Guides

Shamans who perform spiritual healing always have helper spirits who guide them in their healing efforts. What we may attribute to intuition, the Maya attribute to guides. For example, the guide may assist a healer in diagnosing an illness and provide information about the right treatment. The guides also protect the healer from disease, envy, evil spirits, and negative energy.

Every healer has his or her own guides. They can come to the healer in several ways: spontaneous transmission, dream visions, and insight. They can also speak through the sastun.

Just as there are benevolent and malevolent practitioners, there are benevolent and malevolent spirit guides. *Hechiseros,* or "throwers of evil," work with the Nine Malevolent Spirits of the underworld, while the h'men works with Nine Benevolent Spirits of the upper world. Spirit guides are not limited to Maya spirits and can be deities or prophets from other religions.

Ritual and Ceremony

A good healing ritual can make people feel better. Sad to say, the true ritual has pretty much vanished from modern medical practice, unless you consider the ritual of taking an antibiotic before each meal fulfilling. The Maya include ritual in almost every aspect of their healing system. Ritual is fulfilling for both healer and healed. When a healer doesn't know what else to do, a simple ritual of prayer, bathing, and incense can seem close to miraculous. Rituals can also provide closure in times of grief and can help patients to move beyond emotional traumas.

Ceremonies also have tremendous value, especially the Maya *primicia*—the ancient corn ceremony that honors the Maya spirits. When all else fails and the patient is not recovering, h'mens perform the primicia to request assistance from the spirits, especially Ix Chel, the Maya goddess of medicine.

Dream Visions

Dream visions are a tool for guiding and educating healers. They are conduits of ch'ulel at the plane where the physical and spiritual worlds meet. Maya spirits communicate through dreams. Healers tell enchanting tales of nocturnal visits from spirits who appear in various forms and use different methods to instruct.

When confronted with a patient who has confusing symptoms, the Maya healer may say: "I don't really understand your sickness, but I will pray for a dream to help me. You must wait until then."

Most of the time the dream vision comes within a few days, often that very night. Sometimes healers receive a dream before they realize that they haven't completely understood the ailment. A spirit will just show up in a dream and say: "That baby has not only a cough but a lung infection, so you should add this or that plant to the formula and you will get better results."

Incense

Incense is the essence of life, the scent of the spirit. Certain resins and dried parts of sacred plants release ch'ulel when burned. Known mostly as smudging to other Amerindians, the use of incense in medicine is called by the Maya *disafumado,* which in Spanish means "to dispel with smoke." In the sixteenth century a Spanish medical doctor named Bernadino de Sahagun wrote about the frequent use of tree resin as incense in the New World. Around the same time Bernal Diaz, a soldier in Cortez's army, commented in his book *The Conquest of New Spain* on the use of copal in the temples, marketplaces, and homes of the Maya and the Aztec.

The resin of the copal tree is collected with ritual and ceremony on full-moon nights. Bits of copal are dropped on a bed of coals. The copal can be fresh and sticky or dry and brittle. The aroma is unto itself a sacred experience.

Copal is burned for the treatment of all spiritual diseases and considered helpful for many physical ailments. The belief is that the copal incense can rid a person of a harmful or improper thought process, cleanse a home of fear and envy, and act as an offering to the gods and goddesses. Market vendors and shopkeepers burn copal at the beginning of each day to ensure good fortune and dispel envy. Midwives burn copal to give their patients courage during delivery.

In addition to copal, the Maya also burn dried rosemary leaves and powdered balsam bark.

Amulets

Known as *protecciones,* or guards, amulets are much sought after as a means of protecting the wearer against envy, bad luck, and all kinds of negative energy. An amulet can take many forms: Don Elijio made them with balsam bark, a sacred white stone mined from a mountain in Guatemala, copal resin, and fresh rue leaves.

He sewed these ingredients together in a piece of black cloth. Amulets are thought to be powerful purveyors of ch'ulel when they have been blessed by a h'men.

Mano

Mano, or hand in Spanish, is a diagnostic tool. A healer examines the palm for signs of illness or health. Don Elijio liked to study a patient's palm for color, texture, temperature, and response to pressure. Some healers also use mano as a tool of divination.

NOTES

1. David Freidel, Linda Schele, and Joy Parker, *Maya Cosmos: Three Thousand Years on the Shaman's Path* (New York: Morrow, 1993).

2. Daniel Ben Silver, "Zinacanteco Shamanism," Ph.D. dissertation, Harvard University, 1966.

3. Introduction to the Popol Vuh, translated by James A. Fox, Stanford University, at the Poul Vuh Web site: http://www. Stanford.edu/class/anthro98a.

4. Dennis Tedlock, trans., *Popul Vuh: The Mayan Book of the Dawn of Life* (New York: Touchstone/Simon & Schuster, 1985).

5. Tedlock, trans., *Popul Vuh: The Mayan Book of the Dawn of Life.*

6. Freidel, Schele, and Parker, *Maya Cosmos,* p. 51.

7. Sylvanus G. Morley, *The Ancient Maya* (Stanford, CA: Stanford University Press, 1983).

8. Freidel, Schele, and Parker, *Maya Cosmos.*

9. George M. Foster, *Hippocrates' Latin American Legacy: Humoral Medicine in the New World* (Berkeley, CA: Gordon and Breach Science Publishers, 1994).

10. James Boster, *Kekchi Maya Curing Practices in British Honduras* (Cambridge, MA: Harvard University Press, 1973).

11. Silver, "Zinacanteco Shamanism."

12. Boster, *Kekchi Maya Curing Practices.*

13. Foster, *Hippocrates' Latin American Legacy.*

14. Michael Coe, *The Maya,* 1966.

15. Michael Coe, *The Maya.*

16. Freidel, Schele, and Parker, *Maya Cosmos.*

17. Gordon Schendel, *Medicine in Mexico*, 1968.

18. Miriam Chaiken, *Menorahs, Mezuzas, and other Jewish Symbols* (New York: Clarion Books, 1990).

19. Brent and Elois Berlin, *Medical Ethnobotany of the Highland Maya of Chiapas, Mexico: The Gastrointestinal Disease* (Princeton, NJ: Princeton University Press, 1996).

20. Boster, *Kekchi Maya Curing Practices*.

21. Michael Harner, *The Way of the Shaman* (San Francisco: Harper & Row, 1980).

22. Mircea Eliade, *From Medicine Men to Muhammad* (New York: Harper & Row, 1967).

23. Silver, "Zinacanteco Shamanism."

24. Sandra Ingerman, *Soul Retrieval: Mending the Fragmented Self* (San Francisco: HarperSanFrancisco, 1991).

25. Margarita Artschwager Kay, *Healing with Plants in the American and Mexican West* (Tucson: University of Arizona Press, 1996).

26. Bill Gray Douglas, "Illness and Curing in Santiago Atitlan: A Tzutujil Maya Community in the Southwest Highlands of Guatemala," Ph.D. dissertation, Stanford University, 1969).

PART II

Physical Ailments

The Maya healer uses a variety of treatments for physical ailments. Some of the basics are plants and herbs in the form of teas, powders, salves, poultices, and baths, as well as kitchen remedies, massage, diet, and prevention.

This part of the book has five sections: "General Ailments of Adults" is followed by sections on the ailments unique to women, men, and children. Pregnant women should consult a health-care practitioner before consuming medicinal plants in any form or taking hot baths. Look in the women's section under "Childbirth" for home remedies appropriate for use during pregnancy. Adult remedies are not appropriate for children unless otherwise specified.

Many of these remedies make use of medicinal plants that in rare cases may cause an allergic reaction. We suggest that you try this simple skin test before ingesting, applying, or bathing in any of these plants. Apply a few drops of the herbal preparation to the skin at the crease of the inner elbow. Wait five to ten minutes to see whether there is any burning, itching, or swelling. If there is, you may be allergic to that plant and should not take it or use it. For this reason, we always try to include more than one remedy.

A few general pointers:

- *Medicinal plants:* Be sure that any fresh plants you use have not been sprayed with pesticides. Vegetables and fruits should be organic, if possible, for the same reason.
- *Teas:* Always drink a tea before meals. It's easier for you to digest and works better when taken on an empty stomach.
- *Tinctures:* Tinctures are made from medicinal plants that have been steeped in alcohol to extract their active principles. They are more concentrated than herbal teas. One dropperful taken in tepid water is the equivalent of one cup of tea.

- *Powders:* When making powders to apply to the skin, be sure to crush the baked leaves well. Push crushed leaves through a tea strainer to make a fine powder. Remove stems and any large pieces.

General Ailments of Adults

FROM THE KITCHEN

Brown Sugar and Lemon

Combine the juice of one lemon with a teaspoon of brown sugar and mix well. Clean face with soap to remove makeup and lotions. Apply the mixture directly to the face. Let it dry on the face for twenty minutes and then rinse off with tepid water. Repeat twice daily for at least two weeks.

Raw Egg Yolk

Spread raw egg yolk on the face and allow to dry for ten minutes, then wash off with plain water. Repeat this daily for thirty days then twice monthly after that. Repeat occasionally if necessary.

Acne

The Maya never used to have much of a problem with acne, but life has changed for all of us on the planet. So I wasn't surprised when a young Maya woman showed up at my clinic doorstep. She had the worst case of acne I had ever seen. Blood and pus oozed from rivulets in her otherwise beautiful copper-colored face.

She was nineteen and had had acne since she was thirteen. She had tried various prescription medications and over-the-counter anti-acne cream products without success.

Since acne has roots not only in hygiene but in diet, poor eating habits, stress, hormones, toxins, and acids in the blood, I asked her to sit down so that we could talk about her life in general. After a month of the following treatments—and changing her eating habits—this young woman's acne nearly vanished.

Massage The neck and shoulders are areas where many of us hold tension. The resulting tightness of the muscles slows the circulation of blood to and from the face and head, causing stagnation and pooling of impurities. The body tries to eliminate the impurities through the pores, which then become blocked. To relieve the tension and blood stagnation, the Maya healer performs deep muscle massage. For instruction on how to do this massage, see "Ear Infections" in the children's section.

Detox Herbs   To clean the impurities from the blood, take an herbal detox formula daily for ten days, then rest ten days, then repeat. You can purchase one of the wonderful herbal formulas available (see the Resources appendix), or you can make one yourself. Some blood-cleansing herbs—the roots of yellow dock, burdock, and dandelion—are easily found in North America. Try whichever one you can find, and feel free to combine more than one.

ANCIENT WISDOM

Change Your Diet

A diet of simple foods is essential. Eat five servings of fresh, yellow, vitamin A–rich fruits and vegetables daily.

Chew Your Food Properly

Be sure to chew your food thoroughly while it is in your mouth. Properly chewed food digests easily and cuts down on the blood acids that end up coming out through the pores of the skin.

You can take these herbs as teas or tinctures. As a tincture, take one dropper in a half-glass of tepid water before meals three times daily for ten days, rest ten days, then repeat until you see sufficient improvement.

To make a tea, boil a cup of chopped root in a quart of water for ten minutes. If you can't find the fresh roots, a tea can be made by boiling three teaspoons of the dried root powder in three cups of water. Steep the tea for twenty minutes and take one cup before meals three times daily for ten days, rest ten days and repeat as many times as necessary.

Anemia

Anemia causes the same tiredness, dizziness, weakness, and lack of concentration in a Maya village as it does in a London office building. The Maya have many different ways to combat this common ailment, which, when uncomplicated by intestinal parasites, is easy to treat.

In Belize women are expert at making yummy-tasting tonics for anemia. Here are two of my favorites. Both work.

Hibiscus Tonic Red hibiscus flowers are common in some parts of the hemisphere and can be purchased dried as "Flor de Jamaica" at most Spanish grocery stores. They are also available in any supermarket as "Red Zinger" tea.

To make a delicious tonic tea, add half a cup of dried hibiscus flowers and a quarter-teaspoon of powdered cinnamon to a quart of water. Boil together for five minutes and let sit until cool. Add sugar or honey if desired and serve as a table beverage. Nice hot or cold. Kids love it.

Red Clover Tonic Red clover blossoms are "blood builders." They also have a delightful flavor and are found in abundance in the countryside—perhaps even in your own backyard. To prepare a tea of red clover blossoms, fill a quart jar with fresh blossoms between 10:00 A.M. and 3:00 P.M. in order to maximize the nutrients that are drawn up from the roots by the sun. Boil the blossoms with half a teaspoon of cinnamon in two quarts of water for ten minutes, then steep for twenty minutes. Add honey or brown sugar if you wish. Drink one cup (hot or cool) before meals or as a beverage along with meals and snacks. Take this iron- and mineral-rich tea for ten days at a time, then let your body rest and adjust for ten days. Repeat for another ten days if necessary.

Amaranth The Maya prevention strategy is to not only drink teas steeped from dark red-colored plants on a regular basis but to eat dark leafy greens like amaranth. Amaranth is a common plant that grows throughout the Americas from Alaska to Brazil. It may be a weed growing right outside your door; if so, you may have been pulling up a most valuable and historically famous food source of Native Americans. Amaranth is loaded with easy-to-digest iron, minerals, vitamins, and protein. Best of all, it tastes sweet and delicious.

For severe and chronic anemia, I recommend drinking the raw, blended juice. Gather a cup of fresh, healthy amaranth leaves. Wash

FROM THE KITCHEN

Unlike spinach, amaranth greens don't lose their minerals when cooked. Here are a few of my favorite recipes:

Rosita's Italian-Style Amaranth

2 qts fresh amaranth leaves and young stems, washed
2 cloves garlic
1 medium onion
Italian spices
1 can tomato paste
2 Tbsp olive oil
salt and pepper to taste

Steam the amaranth for ten minutes. In the meantime, chop the onion and garlic into small pieces and sauté in the olive oil. When it is well cooked, add the tomato paste until it burns just slightly. Add one cup of water and simmer for ten minutes. Add the amaranth leaves and cook together another five minutes. Serve with brown rice, pasta, mashed potatoes, or corn tortillas and hot spicy salsa.

Asian-Style Amaranth

2 qts fresh amaranth leaves and young stems, washed
¼ c olive oil
2 cloves garlic
1 Tbsp miso (soybean paste)
optional: ½ tsp fresh ginger, grated

Steam the amaranth for ten minutes or boil in a bit of water for five minutes. Blend the rest of the ingredients for one minute. Pour this sauce over the amaranth and toss lightly before serving.

If amaranth greens aren't easily available, substitute collards or kale from your local grocery. Prepare them as for Italian-style or Asian-style amaranth or add them to soups regularly. They are tougher than amaranth, so you will need to boil them for at least thirty minutes first. Even if the kids pick out the leaves, they will benefit from the iron and nutrients infused in the soup.

Fresh Amaranth Broth and Honey

This broth may sound strange, but it is really quite refreshing and good for you. Cool the amaranth stock left in the pot, mix in honey to taste, and drink.

well and place in a blender for a few seconds with a cup of water. Take one-third of a cup of the juice three times daily before meals for ten days, then stop. Rest for ten days and then repeat if needed.

Asthma

We seem to be having a global asthma epidemic, owing perhaps to increasing amounts of pollutants in our air and exacerbated by the stressfulness of our busy modern lives. Overconsumption of dairy products is also a factor.

Asthma is an ailment with a legion of causes. Neither I nor the Maya have an easy solution. But here are some simple home remedies from the Maya that have proven helpful in controlling asthma.

Try these remedies only if you are anticipating an attack or are in the early stages of one. If the asthma progresses, seek medical assistance immediately.

Strong Back The best Maya remedy for adult asthma is a weedy little plant known as strong back. The name comes from its traditional use as a backache remedy. Quite a bit of solid research has been conducted in Africa and Asia on the anti-asthmatic effects of strong back: it relaxes muscle spasms around the chest, eases the flow of mucus, and has a beneficial effect on nerves.

Unless you live in a very warm climate, strong back probably does *not* grow in your backyard. Look in the Resources appendix for places to buy it as a tea or tincture. Strong back is sold in Europe as "Desmodium" in capsule form. Follow the dose instructions on the label. If you are using the tincture, take two droppers in a half-glass of tepid water every twenty minutes until the wheezing stops.

ANCIENT WISDOM
Stay out of Hot and Cold Baths

Maya healers say that asthmatics should never bathe in anything but room-temperature water. Many swear by this idea and use it as a means to control and reduce asthma attacks. Heat tends to increase muscle spasms.

Life Everlasting Life everlasting is another popular antiwheezing remedy. This little plant propagates itself from its own leaves. When a leaf drops to the ground, several new plants sprout from it—thus its name.

Maya healers collect leaves with recently sprouted baby plants growing from them. They mash the sprouted leaves with a pinch of salt, then give the juice by the teaspoonful three times daily. This is said to halt wheezing, ease breathing, and sometimes cure the asthma.

Life everlasting is considered a cure-all by many healers because of its wide range of uses. You can purchase this plant in many nurseries around the world. It is also known by the name mother of thousands. You need only a leaf to start a life everlasting plant in a pot or in the yard. Be sure to bring it indoors during the colder winter months.

Backache

The Maya regularly carry an amazing amount of life's needs on their backs. Men carry wood, bags of cement, and heavy sacks filled with corn and beans. Women carry the same sacks plus children, buckets of water, and laundry to and from the river. This is a culture whose people have far more than their share of backaches.

Strong Back Tea or Tincture Strong back is the herb of choice to be taken orally. I first learned of this wonderful herb while on an ethnobotany expedition in the jungle with the Belizian bushmaster Polo Romero. Every night, after a grueling twelve hours of hard, physical labor, often in the rain and wind, he would brew us a pot of strong back tea. We were all convinced that we would have had backaches if not for his tea.

This plant is little known outside of Central America and the Caribbean but is soon to become famous—mark my words! One reason it is not known is that it can be found only in the tropics. Lucky for us, we live in the age of next-day delivery service, and strong back can be ordered in tincture form (see Resources appendix).

Some Maya healers prescribe strong back in combination with wild yam root for chronic backache.

Purslane Poultice Purslane is a common pan-American weed that grows in gardens, at curbsides, and on doorsteps. It's called *verdalaga* in Spanish. Most folks think of purslane as a pesky weed

FROM THE KITCHEN

Allspice Poultice

Old-timers tell us to boil a small handful of allspice berries or powder in a cup of water until it thickens—about fifteen minutes—then add a pinch of salt. Spread the warm—not hot—mixture on a cloth as for a purslane poultice and apply to the back to relieve pain and inflammation.

and have no idea that they are overlooking a wonderful medicinal herb. I often use this poultice when my back aches from sitting too long at my computer.

Gather the stems and leaves and wash them. Blend them with as little water as possible until the mixture is the consistency of paste. Spread the paste on an old cotton cloth and place over the sore spot on the back. Tie up the poultice with a soft, cotton band or a back belt to hold it in place for a few hours.

The purslane is rich in minerals and calcium that pass through the skin and penetrate into muscle fibers to help them relax. It also alleviates pain, inflammation, and stiffness.

ANCIENT WISDOM

Rapid Temperature Change

Maya people believe that a rapid change in temperature is the cause of many a stiff back and muscle spasm.

One of my patients comes to mind. Linda was a thirty-year-old weightlifting enthusiast who worked out three times a week. She came to see me about her chronic backache. She couldn't figure out why someone as fit and healthy as she was would be having this problem. We talked about her routine for a while, and I discovered that she liked to cool off in front of a fan after every workout.

The Maya would say, "Ooooooh, well, that's why she has a backache!" Cooling off the stretched, warm muscles of her back with a fan caused the cold air to penetrate right through the pores opened by the perspiration, heat, and exercise. The cool air caused the muscles to spasm in response to the rapid change.

Once Linda learned to cool down more gradually—away from the fan—her chronic backache disappeared.

Bladder Infections

Women get bladder infections more often than men. These painful infections are usually caused by improper wiping, which allows *Escherichia coli*—the infamous *E. coli*—from the bowels to find their way into the urinary tract. Diet also plays a role. People who eat a lot of rich food and overeat are more prone to bladder infections.

Bladder infections cause a painful burning sensation and an urgency to urinate. Maya people seek relief by turning to the fields outside their homes. There they find two wonderfully effective remedies. Both act as diuretics and flush out the bacteria from the bladder.

By the way, these remedies are more effective if you avoid carbonated beverages and restrict salt intake, meat, and desserts. A light fare of soup, salad, and fruit is best. Remember to drink at least eight cups of water a day between meals so that the water can act as a flush unimpeded by food.

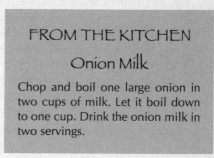

FROM THE KITCHEN

Onion Milk

Chop and boil one large onion in two cups of milk. Let it boil down to one cup. Drink the onion milk in two servings.

If you try these remedies and do not get relief within thirty-six hours, consult a health-care practitioner.

Indian Corn Silk Tea Corn silks are the fine, golden corn hairs that you see every time you shuck an ear of corn. This tea is delicious.

To prepare, collect the hairs of six pieces of corn on the cob. Boil in three cups of water for ten minutes. Steep for thirty minutes and strain. Take in half-cup doses throughout the day. Consume all three cups in one day. Repeat as often as necessary.

Horsetail Tea Horsetail is a lovely, reedlike plant found growing along streams, ponds, and damp areas. When I was younger, I used to collect it along the shores of Lake Michigan. It is available in health food stores. Fresh horsetail can also be dried and stored for the winter.

To prepare, boil a cup of fresh, chopped stems or half a cup of dried leaves and stems in a quart of water for ten minutes. Allow to cool. Strain and sip throughout the day until you have consumed the whole quart.

Bronchitis and Chronic Cough

I have never treated a person suffering from chronic bronchitis or recurrent coughing spells who wasn't also consuming excess amounts of dairy products and experiencing too much daily stress. The combination of mucus-forming foods and a heavy emotional load tightens the chest and clogs the respiratory passages.

Generally these patients have had something bothering them for a long time that they need to "get off their chest." They probably can't be helped until they spill the beans and let go of their fear, anger, or resentment. In most Maya villages men and women readily share their troubles with each other. One of Don Elijio's chief functions in his village of San Antonio was to act as a counselor and sympathetic ear.

Once the emotional weight is lifted, the Maya have some good remedies to help alleviate the *symptoms* of chronic bronchitis and cough.

Oregano and Garlic Tea   The favorite remedy of grannies and healers for bronchitis is oregano and garlic tea. Boil three tablespoons of dried oregano and three cloves of chopped garlic *with skins* in a quart of water for ten minutes. Steep for five minutes.

Cautiously bend your head over the steaming pot, wrap a towel around your head and neck to keep the steam in, and breathe deeply for five minutes. Take care not to get a steam burn. If the steam feels painful to the skin on your face, it is too hot. Repeat the steam treatment as needed to speed relief. Try this treatment before bedtime. It promotes sound sleep and is good for kids too.

Drink the tea itself in half-cup doses every two hours throughout the day. Add honey and lime juice before serving if desired.

Onion Juice and Honey   Blend half an onion, two teaspoons of honey, and one teaspoon of fresh grated ginger for twenty seconds. Take two tablespoons after dinner daily as needed.

FROM THE KITCHEN
All-Purpose Maya Cough Syrup

Cough syrups, known as *jarebes,* are popular among the Maya. Most healers make them ahead of time so that they are ready to dispense as needed. You can make an excellent cough syrup right in your own kitchen. Be sure to include the kids. It's a fun project, and they'll beg you for a taste of the sweet-tasting medicine.

2 Tbsp fresh ginger, grated
3 cloves garlic, chopped with skins
2 Tbsp dried oregano
2 Tbsp dried lemongrass or anise seeds
1 qt water
2 c brown sugar
juice of 1 lemon

Boil the ginger, garlic, oregano, and lemongrass in the water over medium heat in a covered glass or porcelain pot for thirty minutes. Strain and add sugar and lemon juice.

Dose: Adults and children over six can take one tablespoon every hour. Children between three and six should take one teaspoon every hour.

Nighttime variation: For a nighttime cough syrup, add two tablespoons of dried vervain leaves or one tablespoon of dried vervain root to the formula. Take at bedtime. If you can't get vervain, use two tablespoons of chamomile, melissa (also known as lemon balm), or passionflower.

Vervain Tea For the cough that is worse at night, drink a strong cup of tea made from vervain about an hour before retiring.

To prepare, boil one entire plant of vervain or half a cup of dried vervain in three cups of water for ten minutes. Steep for twenty minutes. Drink as hot as possible. Don't add honey for flavor because it may be stimulating and prevent sleep. Keep a thermos of the prepared warm tea at your bedside for easy access during the night.

Bruises

"Ouch! I really hurt myself today falling down the stairs," said the voice on the other end of the telephone. "What can I do? My right foot is swollen and black and blue."

FROM THE KITCHEN
Lemon for Bruises

Recently I took a group of pharmacy students into the rainforest to see the unexcavated mound of an ancient Maya temple. I took a shortcut to the top, and even though I knew the rocks were loose, I placed all my weight on a pile, which gave out from under me. I fell with all my weight onto my left thigh, jamming it into a sharp rock. The bruise was the worst I have ever had—big as a grapefruit and black, blue, yellow, and red.

When I got back to Ix Chel Farm, the traditional Maya healer Beatrice Waight was there. She went into our kitchen and came out with a lemon. She sliced it in half and rubbed the lemon pulp over my bruise, directing me to repeat this throughout the day every hour or so. My bruise improved quickly. Lemon reduces swelling, and vitamin C promotes healing.

The answer was easy. I knew the caller—my friend Isabella—and I knew that she had a healthy and vigorous oregano plant growing in her garden. I told her how to make the following tea.

Isabella called me a few days later singing the praises of the oregano plant that had helped her so much.

"Who would have thought it!" she exclaimed. "Something so simple and growing right there in my garden all the time. Wonderful!"

Oregano Tea Bath Cut off three 12-inch branches (or use three tablespoons of dried leaves) and boil them in two quarts of water for twenty minutes. When the tea has cooled, soak your bruise in it for thirty minutes twice daily. You can also soak a cotton cloth in the oregano tea and wrap it around the bruise to wear throughout the day.

Burns (Minor Only)

During the early years on our farm in Belize we had an old wood cookstove in our palm-thatch kitchen. One day, while standing at the stove, I was surprised by a visitor who seemed to come out of nowhere. I turned and knocked a pot of boiling water onto my leg.

It was a nasty, deep burn, and it started to get infected. Mr. Thomas Green—a famous ninety-three-year-old Creole healer who lives a few miles up the river—came by in his canoe to visit.

When he saw my burn, he walked into the garden and came back with a handful of oregano and eggplant leaves.

"Boil these up good, and when the water cools off, use it to wash your leg several times a day," he explained. "Just use a cup and pour the cooled tea over the burn."

Well! Even I was surprised to see how quickly the burn began to heal. After the first bath the infection seemed to gather itself together and dry up. By the third day the burn was well on its way to healing. Pink, healthy skin was growing over the burn. Mr. Thomas later said that tomato leaves with oregano would have worked as well.

QUICK RELIEF
Aloe

Aloe vera has been famous as a healing agent since biblical times. Cut a fresh piece and slice off the ends and prickly sides. Scoop out the inner jelly with a spoon and rub directly on the burn several times daily. The aloe is very cooling and prevents scarring.

Burns are easily infected, so take care to keep them clean with a sterile pad and change it frequently. Use common sense. If a burn is serious, large, or blistered, get help.

FROM THE KITCHEN
Sunburn Remedy

Here is an emergency treatment for sunburn that is easy to get anywhere, anytime. Steep six regular black tea bags in six cups of hot water for fifteen minutes to release their tannins—the astringents that help alleviate inflammation and pain. Refrigerate the tea bags in the tea water until they are nice and cool. Place the tea bags over the sunburn like a poultice and replace every twenty minutes with more cold tea bags. Repeat three times a day or as often as necessary.

The cold liquid tea can also be poured over the burn or used to soak a burned foot or hand. Soak for twenty minutes and refrigerate the tea water again for use later.

Oregano and Eggplant (or Tomato) Leaves Boil a large handful (about two cups) of oregano and eggplant (or tomato) leaves in a gallon of water for ten minutes. When the water cools, wash the burn with a quart of the liquid. Repeat frequently throughout the day.

Desert Nopal The classic Maya burn remedy, the desert nopal, is extremely effective.

Since the desert nopal is a cactus with small thorns, wear gloves when you collect it. Use a knife to scrape off the almost invisible thorns. Slice it in half, then use the knife to loosen and scrape the inner gel and rub that over the burn several times a day for quick relief of pain and prevention of blisters.

The desert nopal can be found in the southern and western regions of the United States. Also a food, nopal is sold fresh in some grocery stores. Dried nopal can be found in Spanish grocery stores. Boil one small package of the dried nopal in a quart of water for twenty minutes. When cool, wash the burn. You can reboil the same nopal a second time.

Here are two other burn remedies from the kitchen and garden that also work. Use whichever is more convenient.

Raw Potato Clean the burn with cold water and then apply a slice of raw potato immediately. Lightly wrap the potato to the burn. Change the potato every half-hour for a day.

Banana Leaf Poultice I once visited a hospital burn unit in Guatemala City. I was thrilled to see that all the patients had banana leaves wrapped around their burns. When I asked a nurse why they used banana leaves, she shrugged and said nonchalantly, "Because they are the best for treating second- and third-degree burns. We change them twice a day and wash the wounds in between. The banana leaves prevent blistering."

Carpal Tunnel Syndrome

I now have a computer at my farm in Belize, and lo and behold, I recently began to feel those pains in my wrist that I had heard so much about. Carpal tunnel syndrome is caused by pressure on the nerve that passes from the spinal column, over the shoulders, down the wrist, and finally to the hands. The usual symptoms are pain, tingling, and stiffness of the wrist and fingers.

Using what I know of Maya treatments, I came up with the following remedies. They are similar to what Don Elijio and his friends used back in the days when their wrists ached from wielding machetes.

I heated some olive oil, then massaged it very deeply into the flesh between my elbow and wrist. Wow! I was shocked to feel some excruciatingly painful spots, but I just kept right on, stopping every few minutes to pinch the flesh between my thumb and forefinger to let the congestion move out of the area and into general circulation.

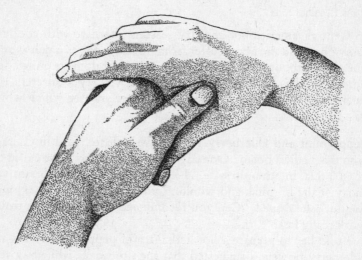

I took the rest of the day off and was back at the computer the next day able to put in another six hours pain-free. I repeated the elbow-to-wrist massage once each day for a week. I now use this remedy occasionally in order to prevent another flare-up.

Cabbage Leaf Poultice A poultice of common cabbage leaves mashed up with castor oil (olive oil works too) is an effective herbal treatment for carpal tunnel syndrome. Pick one or two of the greenest outer leaves from the plant or the cabbage head. Blend the leaves with the castor oil until it forms a thick paste.

Spread the paste on a piece of old cotton and heat it in the microwave or a steamer until it's above body temperature. (Don't burn yourself, and don't do this if you have diabetes because you might not be able to feel the heat.) Lay the paste and cotton on the skin between the elbow and wrist. Wrap up the cotton with a kitchen towel and rest your arm on a heating pad set on low heat for twenty minutes.

The mustard oil in the cabbage leaves acts as a decongestant and improves the circulation of blood, lymph, and nerve. If you are allergic to mustard oil, don't do this treatment. Use fresh Saint-John's-wort instead.

Colds and Flu

In Central America hot and dry seasons alternate with cool and rainy ones, and the Maya suffer from flu and colds as much as anyone else. Although they have no "cures," they do have quite a few home remedies that are logical and effective. Try a different one each time you're feeling under the weather and see which works best for you.

Peppermint and Elderberry Tea   I have a close friend in Chicago who is a medical doctor. One day while I was in town she called me at 6:00 A.M. in a frantic state. "I have to deliver an important talk today at the hospital, and wouldn't you know it, I woke up with the flu," she rasped. "Can you recommend something that would work really fast?"

I told her to prepare a hot herbal tea of peppermint leaves and elderberry flowers. I suggested that she sip the tea while in a very hot bath, then get into bed and cover her body and head with warm covers. Once there she was to put a hot water bottle or heating pad to her feet and sweat.

She called me back later that day, elated. Her flu symptoms had vanished. She delivered her talk that afternoon feeling strong and healthy.

Increasing the body temperature by several degrees brings on an artificial fever that destroys viruses and cleanses toxic waste from the body. Together the elderberry and peppermint stimulate perspiration and fight the virus.

FROM THE GARDEN
Herbal Bath

Another wonderful Maya remedy is a hot bath with marigold flowers and leaves, followed by a cup of hot peppermint tea with lemon and honey. Afterward wrap up warm and go to sleep.

To prepare the marigold bath, boil six large stems (about twelve inches long) with flower heads and leaves in two gallons of water in your largest pot for ten minutes. Strain and pour into a tub of hot water. Test the temperature of the bath to avoid scalding. Soak yourself for twenty minutes. When you're out of the bath, wrap up your head with a towel or woolen cap, put on a pair of wool socks and pajamas, pull up your warmest covers, sip on the hot peppermint tea, and allow yourself to sweat it out. This really works!

Caution: Take only *warm* herbal bath soaks if you are pregnant or have high blood pressure, low blood pressure, asthma, heart trouble, or diabetes. The water should be only slightly above body temperature.

Garlic, Cayenne, and Jackass Bitters Tincture One of my favorite cold and flu remedies is a combination of garlic, cayenne pepper, and jackass bitters. Where jackass bitters is not available, echinacea is a good substitute. These plants are strongly antiviral and antimicrobial expectorants.

At home I plan ahead by combining a whole head of chopped garlic (skins and all) with a teaspoonful of cayenne pepper and a cup of jackass bitters leaves (or three tablespoons of echinacea powder) into a quart of rum. I let it soak for ten days, away from the sun. When I need it, I take this concentrated tincture by the teaspoonful with honey, juice, or water.

If the cold is caught early enough, one dose can chase it away within hours. If the cold is a day old, take three large tablespoons throughout the day. If you've had the cold for a few days, it may take longer to get rid of it. This has been my household remedy for decades. I call it "Flu-Away" (see Resources appendix).

Lemon Juice and Honey This is great for kids. Squeeze the juice of one lemon into a glass and add a tablespoon or two of honey and

hot water. Drink three glasses in sips throughout the day before
meals and at bedtime. The combination of honey and lemon is
antimicrobial, expectorant, soothing to the throat, and relaxing.
The vitamin C in the lemons is easily absorbed by the body and
helps beef up your immune system and cell function. Limes work
just as well.

Hot Ginger Tea Hot ginger tea sipped throughout the day stimulates circulation, helping to loosen mucus from the lungs and
sinuses and warm the body.

   Grate three tablespoons of fresh ginger and boil for five minutes
in three and a half cups of water. Steep covered for ten minutes and

FROM THE KITCHEN
Sick People Soup

When you have a cold or the flu, the best strategy is to drink plenty of fluids—water, hot teas, juices, and soups. Avoid all dairy products, white
rice, and white bread because they increase phlegm and discourage elimination. Here's a recipe for the common cold that my family calls "Sick
People Soup":

$1/2$ head cabbage, chopped
1 onion, chopped
1 head garlic, chopped
3 carrots, sliced
3 pieces celery, diced
6 Tbsp ginger, grated
$1/4$ c miso (soybean paste)
2 qts water
juice of 1 lemon or lime

   Boil the vegetables in the water until tender (about thirty minutes),
then add ginger and garlic and allow to boil another five minutes.
Remove from heat. Take a bit of the hot soup from the pot and mix with
the miso to form a thick liquid. Add to the soup and serve. Squeeze a bit
of fresh lime juice into the bowl. For an added health boost, sprinkle
crushed garlic on the soup before serving.
   Miso can be purchased in health food stores everywhere.

drink as hot as possible. You may add honey. Ginger has antiviral compounds and gingerol—an essential oil that stimulates perspiration, reduces fever, and loosens phlegm.

Pregnant women should avoid ginger because it may stimulate too much circulation to the uterus and cause a miscarriage.

Onion, Garlic, and Honey Soak one chopped onion and one head of garlic in two pints of honey overnight. Eat only the honey by the teaspoonful several times daily. The onions and garlic contain sulfur and other germicidal compounds long known around the world as powerful cold fighters. Eating raw onions and garlic during the winter months is a good preventive measure against the contagious common cold.

Constipation

Until the last few decades constipation was almost unknown among the Maya. Their high-fiber diet of corn, beans, and pumpkins was supplemented by garden vegetables and seasonal fruits. Since the arrival of soft drinks and processed foods, however, constipation has become common.

A good diet, a daily walk, at least three pieces of fruit daily (try ripe mangoes!), and at least eight glasses a day of plain water are the best prevention. Follow the FEW principle—Fiber, Exercise, and Water. But when you are stuck and need action, try one of the Maya's intestinal purges.

Although I don't share the Central American obsession with purging, these natural remedies do work wonders. They also help in treating common ailments such as fevers, skin conditions, headaches, and acne. Of course, don't overdo laxatives. You don't want to become dependent on them. Purges also are not for pregnant women.

If you don't see improvement, consult your health-care practitioner. There may be some other reason for your constipation.

Aloe Vera Purge Good old aloe vera is just about everyone's favorite. We take it raw and juiced. To make aloe juice, cut two 8- to 10-inch pieces from the plant and wash well. Don't remove the aloe skin. Blend the aloe with just enough water to facilitate the blending action. Drink it all up on an empty stomach about half an hour before a meal. Within twelve hours you should have a copious, soft, and comfortable bowel movement that may be preceded by minor stomach cramping.

Aloe vera capsules are available at stores that sell health foods. Take two capsules and you will have an urgent but comfortable bowel movement in about eight hours' time.

Castor Oil and Orange Juice For fast and sure results, good old-fashioned castor oil with orange juice is the treatment of choice for most Maya people. The castor tree grows abundantly throughout Central America.

Mix one tablespoon with four ounces of OJ for adults and children over twelve. Drink on an empty stomach about half an hour before eating. For younger children mix one teaspoon with four ounces of orange juice. Do not give to children under the age of four (see "Purges" in the section on children's ailments).

Cuts and Scrapes

For nine years I was part of a team of collectors who combed the rainforests of Belize for plants to send to the National Cancer Institute. The NCI then tested these plants for anti-cancer and anti-AIDS activity. This was dangerous, hard work, and we frequently cut or scraped ourselves in the process. Sometimes our cuts got infected. Here are some of my favorite tried-and-true remedies for minor cuts and scrapes.

QUICK RELIEF
Aloe Vera Remedy

Scrape out the inside gel and apply to the wound. Some people cut open pieces of aloe and tie them around the cut with the slimy side down against the skin.

By the way, the leaves of the following plants can be reduced to a juicy pulp by chewing or blending. Be sure to check the leaves for insects and rinse them off in clean water. It is best if the person who has the cut does the chewing. Place the pulp over the cut or scrape and hold it in place with a clean cloth or handkerchief. Always wash the cut or scrape with clean water and soap first.

Amaranth: works well to stop bleeding
Basil: prevents infection and speeds healing
Red clover (leaves or flowers): stops bleeding, pain, and infection

FROM THE KITCHEN
Wound Powder

For more serious cuts and wounds, prepare this wound powder ahead of time and store it in a glass jar. It will last a full three years as long as it is protected from mold.

$\frac{1}{2}$ c fresh basil leaves
$\frac{1}{2}$ c red clover leaves
$\frac{1}{2}$ c marigold leaves
$\frac{1}{2}$ c amaranth leaves

Wash well and remove insects. Let dry on a towel for half an hour. Place on a cookie sheet in a slow oven (200 degrees) until crispy dry (about forty-five minutes).

Crumble and remove stems and leaf veins. Place in a dry skillet over medium heat and stir constantly with a wooden spoon until the plant parts are actually burning. They should get very dark and smoky. The burning is necessary to release the minerals and healing ingredients in the ash of the plants. When the leaves are well toasted, pass them through a sieve to reduce them to a fine powder. Discard all of the denser pieces left in the strainer. Don't forget to label and date the jar.

Sprinkle the powder over clean wounds that have been moistened with a few drops of castor oil.

Diarrhea

People tend to identify Central America with diarrhea, thanks in part to the old joke about Montezuma's revenge. Fortunately, the Maya happen to have quite a few good methods of staving off "revenge."

Of course, acute diarrhea can be a good thing—the body is try-ing to eliminate something that might be harmful if absorbed into the system. So the Maya first give the diarrhea a chance to do its job before they halt the process. You can do the same, but don't let it go for more than twenty-four hours and be sure to replace your fluid loss by drinking lots of water and electrolyte supplements (available at most stores in the juice section), which replace vital nutrients.

The problem with some over-the-counter antidiarrhea medications is how abruptly they halt the elimination of poisons. Herbal alternatives act more slowly and provide the added benefit of destroying the bacteria or amoebas right in the stomach and bowel while giving the body time to rid itself of unwanted material.

Red Hibiscus Flowers and Cinnamon Tea   This is an easy and effective first-aid remedy for diarrhea. If red hibiscus is not available, try pink or red hollyhock flowers. Boil nine flowers and half a teaspoon of cinnamon in two cups of water for five minutes, steep until cool, strain, and take in half-cup doses every hour.

Red Rose Tea   If you don't have hibiscus or hollyhock, pick a few red roses. Choose only roses that you know have not been sprayed with pesticides or herbicides.

Boil three red roses, each with six inches of leaves and stems, in three cups of water for ten minutes. Steep tea until cooled to room temperature. Take half a cup every two hours throughout the day. Repeat for two to three days if necessary. You may add half a teaspoon of powdered cinnamon if desired.

Dry Skin

Our skin dries out for many reasons. Most of the time dry skin is due to insufficient water intake, too little oil or fat in the diet, or nervousness.

Stress and anxiety cause dry skin because, as the muscles tighten in response to the tension, the blood supply to the skin is diminished, leaving it with insufficient nutrients to maintain optimum skin moisture. Walking, stretching, and yoga can counteract this effect. Nerve-calming teas made from linden flowers, chamomile, or man vine from the rainforest also work well. Other relaxants found in a convenient tincture form are passionflower and kava kava. Take as directed on the label.

I always get dry skin when I travel. The environments of airplanes, hotels, and conference halls are dehydrating. To counteract this effect, I drink plenty of water—three quarts a day—and bring along a small bottle of olive oil to use on my skin and to take internally—just one teaspoon a day helps.

Other good sources of oil are the essential fatty acids in nuts and seeds. Sesame seeds are the Maya choice. They roast the raw seeds on their clay *comals*, grind them into a meal, and add the sesame to corn to make delicious cakes and crackers.

Among the many good sources of sesame are Middle Eastern halvah candy and tahini (sesame paste), both available at all health food stores. Tahini can be added to salads and steamed vegetables and mixed into sautéed vegetables.

FROM THE KITCHEN

Toasted Sesame Seed Salsa

1 c raw sesame seeds, cleaned
1 large tomato or 1 small can stewed tomatoes
2 cloves garlic
cayenne pepper and salt to taste

Place sesame seeds in dry frying pan over low heat, stirring constantly with a wooden spoon until the seeds begin to jump out of the pan. When they are cool, grind them in a coffee or seed grinder. If using a fresh tomato, boil in a bit of water until soft. Remove the skin. Place tomato, garlic, sesame, cayenne, and salt in a blender for one minute, adding water if necessary to achieve a creamy consistency. Serve with soft or hard tortillas, over salad, or over brown rice.

Fainting

My daughter was a fainter from the ages of eleven through sixteen. It wasn't easy to discover the real problem. Caused by a sudden loss of oxygen to the brain, fainting can be a sign of anemia, heart trouble, hypoglycemia, or the early stages of pregnancy. It can be brought on by hunger, stuffy rooms, extreme pain, shock, or trauma. Repeated fainting can be a sign of something serious and needs to be brought to the attention of a medical doctor.

Try as we might, we could find no metabolic reason for Crystal's fainting bouts. She was finally diagnosed with nonmetabolic hypoglycemia brought on by emotional upsets. We gave her relaxing teas such as chamomile, linden flowers, and melissa, which helped a great deal. We also learned how to be better parents.

When someone feels faint, place the head between the legs—this quickly brings oxygen and blood to the brain. If the person has already fainted, doing the same will bring him or her back to consciousness. Here are several other suggestions straight from the Maya tradition.

Rue Rub   Maya healers always keep a preparation made of rue leaves and rubbing alcohol on hand to rub on the forehead and palms of a person who has fainted. Be careful not to get the rue into the eyes, mouth, or nose. The rue stimulates blood flow to the brain. Healers also soak a cotton ball in the preparation and place it under the nostrils of someone who is about to faint. The aroma stimulates blood circulation.

Making the preparation is easy. Purchase a pint bottle of rubbing alcohol and add nine 6-inch branches of fresh rue leaves with, if possible, flowers. Don't worry if no flowers are available—the leaves will do the job. Steep the rue in the alcohol for three days before using. Keep handy but out of the reach of children.

Aromatic Herbs   Crushing aromatic herbs to place under the nose of a fainter is the equivalent of "smelling salts." Basil, rosemary, sage, or oregano work well. So do orange leaves.

Fever

One day, when my daughter was nine, she developed a sudden fever of 102 degrees. A traditional healer was staying at our farm, and when I asked her for assistance, she didn't bother to treat the fever. Instead, she administered a purge from a common variety of the senna bush known as Christmas candle. Its name stems from the tall, bright yellow blossoms that bloom in December.

Within an hour Crystal had a copious bowel movement and the fever went down. Later that day the fever rose again, and the healer prepared a lovely-tasting tea made from lemongrass. (Add a bit of honey and this tea tastes like candy.) Crystal soon felt better and was less feverish. We gave her two more cups during the afternoon. That night she sweated so much that we had to change her sheets twice. By five o'clock the next morning she was hungry and ready to go out and play.

I have learned from the Maya not to be afraid of fevers. They are Mother Nature's way of fighting invading organisms, and she needs time to do her thing. Fever fights off infection, invaders, and viruses by raising the body's temperature and activating the immune system. The foreign organisms cannot survive the higher temperature.

Fever provides toxins with the opportunity to exit the bloodstream. So if you stop a fever too soon, the immune system doesn't have the time it needs to "houseclean." Obviously there is a limit to how high and long you should let a fever run. Generally, if a fever rises above 102 degrees Fahrenheit, seek medical advice. If unconsciousness or convulsions accompany the fever, see a doctor immediately.

A good first step in managing a fever is to administer a laxative. Any of the laxatives listed under "Constipation" will help to reduce the fever.

Fever-Reducing Teas Most aromatic plants with essential oils reduce fevers by increasing perspiration, which both cools the body and lets toxins out through the sweat glands. Try basil, rosemary, thyme, ginger, oregano, lemongrass, or sage. Choose whichever one is most appealing and convenient.

Aromatic Herb Formula Boil three tablespoons of any of the dried herbs above with three cups of water for five minutes. (If using fresh lemongrass, you need six leaves.) Steep covered for ten minutes. Drink as hot as possible, keep warm in bed, and sweat it out.

Fungus

There is lots of fungus among us in the tropics! Necessity is the mother of invention, and the Maya have come up with impressive antifungal treatments. Also, Nature provides for her own: the tropics are home to some plants with powerful antifungal properties.

A few years back a young Maya mother of four took me aside in the marketplace in the nearby town of San Ignacio. She asked what I could recommend for skin fungus, then raised up her blouse to show me a ring of weeping, crusty fungus around her waist.

It is not unusual to find fungal infections where the body perspires regularly. The waist, back of the neck, feet, underarms, and buttocks are common sites.

Fortunately for this Maya mother, the very plant she needed was growing only a few feet away from us along the bank of the Macal River. I love it when this happens.

"Do you know this plant?" I asked her.

"Sure! That's the *tres puntas*, isn't it?"

"Right! It is also known as jackass bitters. That's the plant you need, *mamasita.*"

The jackass bitters worked like a charm. When next I saw her, she was bending over a bin of coconuts at the market. She looked up, smiled, and reported that the fungus was healed but that she still kept the tres puntas on hand in the shower for prevention.

FROM THE KITCHEN

Allspice Ointment for Foot Fungus

This recipe comes from Don Elijio's teacher, Jeronimo Requena, bush-doctor to the intrepid *chicleros* in the 1920s. The chicleros lived long months in the damp jungles extracting chicle, which was used as the base for gum (thus the name "Chiclets"). Foot fungus was an occupational hazard for chicleros.

Mix one teaspoon of powdered allspice with three teaspoons of vegetable shortening and combine into a paste. Apply to the affected area three times daily. This works best on *dry* foot fungus.

Jackass bitters is absolutely the best plant I have *ever* encountered for treating skin fungus or athlete's foot. It does not grow in temperate climes, but you can order it (see the Resources appendix).

Jackass bitters works great on foot fungus. Not long ago one of my employees came to see me in the early morning hours to say he could not work that day because his feet were too sore.

"What's the problem?" I asked.

"Look at this," he said as he removed his rubber boots and nylon socks.

I took a deep breath when I saw that foot fungus had eaten holes in his heels the width of a pencil. The holes were a half-inch or so deep. It was awful. I couldn't imagine how this man had managed to work the previous days. Foot soaks of jackass bitters and switching to cotton socks did wonders for him.

Jackass Bitters Tea Boil a cup of the dried leaves in two quarts of water for twenty minutes and bathe the area several times daily or apply with cotton swabs and air-dry.

To treat feet, prepare the tea in the same way and soak the foot in it twice daily, in the morning and in the evening. Soak the appropriate part of cotton socks in the same solution and wear them all day. Repeat for three weeks if necessary.

Garlic Toenail Fungus Remedy Trim your toenails, then run the file across the entire length of the nail from tip to cuticle. Push the cuticle back to expose the skin around the nail. (Don't use these nail tools again without sterilizing them with alcohol.)

Peel and cut in half a clove of garlic and rub it back and forth for a few minutes several times a day over the nail and cuticle. Sometimes this remedy gets rid of the nail fungus within weeks. It may take months, but be diligent and you will get results. If raw garlic is too much for you, purchase odor-free garlic oil capsules. Break them open and apply with a cotton swab at least three times daily. Wear freshly laundered cotton socks after each treatment.

Gallstones

These form in the gall bladder when bile from the liver and cholesterol produce hard, stonelike substances that cause intense pain when they clog the common bile duct. Gallstone pain has become a frequent ailment among the Maya, probably owing to recent dietary changes.

One day a neighbor stopped me on the street and asked whether there was any Maya remedy that could help her daughter get rid of gallstones.

"The doctors say they can't operate because she just had surgery a few weeks ago, and anyway, she doesn't want to lose her gall bladder if there is another way," she explained.

As she spoke, I remembered an old potter in Mexico who had taught me this secret for painlessly passing gallstones. This remedy is common to other cultures as well. Try this only if you have already been diagnosed with gallstones.

Gallstone-Passing Regime Eat no food after lunch. Drink a quart of room-temperature apple juice throughout the afternoon. At

6:00 P.M. set out a cup of olive oil and a cup of fresh lemon juice. Take a teaspoon of each every fifteen minutes until you are nauseous. Then drink a strong cup of chamomile tea (three tea bags to one cup or two tablespoons of the dried herb) that is as hot as you can bear and go to bed. You will awaken during the night to defecate. You will also probably defecate again the next morning.

In your stools you will see greenish round balls—these are the gallstones. Repeat after six weeks' time if you wish to make sure that all the stones have passed.

Gallstone Prevention The Maya take one tablespoon of olive oil plus one tablespoon of lemon juice every morning before breakfast three to five times a week.

Gingivitis

If your gums are swollen and red and bleed easily and your teeth are loose, you have the symptoms of gum disease. Bacteria that deposit plaque on the gums are thought to be the culprit. Here's a Maya treatment that has given me good results. If the symptoms don't go away, see your dentist.

Maya Mouthwash Boil one tablespoon of dried chamomile flowers (or a quarter-cup of fresh blossoms) in a cup of water for five minutes. Steep for twenty minutes. Strain well and mix with one 3-inch piece of aloe vera or one tablespoon of aloe vera juice and one-eighth of a teaspoon of cayenne pepper.

Rinse your mouth with this mouthwash twice daily. Brush and floss regularly. If using fresh aloe, refrigerate.

Gout

Ouch! Just saying the word *gout* makes me cringe. Gout is a painful condition that primarily affects men over the age of thirty. Uric acid crystals accumulate in the joints, causing inflammation, pain, and redness. Usually the first sign of gout is a chronically red, swollen, throbbing, sensitive big toe. The pain is worse when standing.

Gout used to be known as the "rich man's disease" because excess uric acid can be caused by eating rich, protein-laden, creamy foods and drinking wine and beer with meals.

Herbs can eliminate and break down uric acid crystals so that they do not accumulate. The Maya prescribe blood-purifying herbs such as China root and Mexican wild yam. North American blood purifiers are yellow dock, burdock, and dandelion. These are available—often combined in a formula—at most health food stores in tincture, tea, or capsule form.

Whatever you do, don't forget to exercise and eat simple, wholesome foods.

China Root and Wild Yam Tincture Take four droppers of a mix of China root and wild yam daily in a quart of water. Sip all day.

> ## ANCIENT WISDOM
>
> ### Gout Foot Rub
>
> Maya healers prescribe long bare-foot walks on stony paths to stimulate circulation in gouty feet. A glass bottle or foot roller works just as well. Firmly roll your foot back and forth for five minutes twice a day.

China Root and Wild Yam Tea Boil a small handful of China root and wild yam in three cups of water for ten minutes. Strain and drink before meals.

Hangover

It's too bad that the Maya know as much about hangovers as they do. Don Elijio himself was a heavy drinker for many of his 103 years. Indeed, when his wife Chinda died, he nearly drank himself to death. He used to tell lots of stories about his drinking days. One recurrent theme was Chinda's treatment for his hangovers.

Chinda's Favorite Hangover Remedy Boil the rind from one medium-sized orange or twelve orange tree leaves in one quart of water for ten minutes. Remove the rinds and leaves from the water. Add half a cup of cornmeal (the Maya use fresh-ground corn), a pinch of salt, and one tablespoon of brown sugar to the water and continue boiling over low heat until the mixture is thick and smooth. Drink one cup as hot as possible every half-hour until the pot is empty.

This remedy encourages urination and perspiration, helping to cleanse the alcohol from the body. Don Elijio said it worked beautifully. By early afternoon he was usually back in his cornfield, feeling quite chipper.

Epazote Remedy for *Crudo* I spent seven years in the state of Guerrero in southern Mexico, where they call hangovers *crudo*. In Spanish, *crudo* means raw.

> 1 entire plant of epazote (Mexican wormseed)
> 1 qt water
> pinch of salt

Wash the plant well and boil the salt, root, stems, and leaves of the epazote in the quart of water for ten minutes. Drink a cup as hot as possible every half-hour until the pot is empty. Epazote, considered a weed, is found in both tropic and temperate climates.

Headaches

ANCIENT WISDOM

Normalizing Blood Circulation

It helps to pinch and squeeze the soft flesh between the thumb and forefinger while waiting for a poultice to take effect. This helps to normalize the blood circulation to the brain. Acupuncturists know this as the "large intestine four point," which treats pain and encourages drainage in the face.

Headaches are the most prevalent complaint among the Maya, owing perhaps to overexposure to the sun and the stress of daily life. Common headaches can be caused by tension, constipation, allergic reactions, dehydration, hormonal fluctuations, indigestion, and anemia. The natural alternatives to aspirin and pain killers developed by the Maya are very effective treatments. The Maya especially like to use a variety of plants to make poultices, which work as well as aspirin or even better.

Desert Nopal Desert nopal leaf pads are the poultice of choice. Wear thick gloves to remove the leaf pad from the plant because of the almost invisible thorns. With a knife scrape off the thorns and slice open the pad into two pieces. Loosen the gel inside and place the pad on the forehead. Tie it up with a scarf or cloth and keep it there for half an hour. The headache should start to feel better in about ten minutes. The Maya believe that the cactus draws excess heat out of the head.

Hibiscus Another plant poultice is made from the red or pink flowering hibiscus plants. If you can't locate fresh hibiscus, red or pink hollyhocks will work as well. Take nine of the open flowers and nine of the leaves. Mash in a basin with half a cup of water until you have a thick, slimy goo. Spread the goo on a piece of cotton cloth and place the cloth on your forehead. Hold in place with a bandanna or torn strips of sheets. Lie down for an hour if possible.

> ## FROM THE KITCHEN
> ### Ginger for Headaches
> I've seen Central American people carry a bit of fresh ginger around with them to ward off headaches. Whether at work or on the run, they chew a piece of ginger for about half an hour. It can be made into a hot tea. Inhale the steam from the cup while drinking.

Maya Migraine Remedy You will need some equipment: a basin large enough for both feet, a kettle of hot water, a bucket of cold water, a medium-sized towel, and one ounce of brandy.

Place your feet in a basin of hot water, adding more from a kettle at your side as it cools off. Soak the towel in a bucket of cold tap water, wring it out, and place it around your head and neck. Repeat every five minutes to maintain a cool temperature. If dramatic improvement does not take place in ten minutes, sip an ounce of brandy. Always pinch the area between the thumb and forefinger. This treatment lasts thirty minutes.

Note: If you are diabetic, you will need someone to check the temperature of the hot water for you.

Teas Other popular home remedies from south of the border are hot teas of lemongrass, basil, allspice, peppermint, thyme, or oregano.

Chamomile tea is very helpful for tension headaches, especially for children.

High Blood Pressure

Thom was a red-faced Vietnam War veteran suffering from classic postwar trauma. While vacationing in Belize, he came to my clinic at Ix Chel Farm to see whether there was some herbal remedy he could take for his high blood pressure, which could often soar to 190 over 110.

I suggested he cut down on salt, fat, meat, and highly processed foods and that he drink more water. Then I made the following recommendations based on what I have learned from Central American healers.

Chayote Chayote is a tropical fruit from a backyard vine, known also as cho-cho and vegetable pear. It is readily available in most markets that sell Spanish foods. Chayote clears the arteries of plaque. Belizian healers boil it with the skin still on and add a few cloves of garlic to serve as a vegetable dish. It can also be eaten raw or grated on salads or added to soup.

Papaya Papaya is a common backyard garden food grown by most rural families in Central America. My Maya friends tell me that they eat it daily as a snack or after meals to lower blood pressure. Papaya has many wonderful healing properties. It's even better for you with a generous squeeze of fresh lime or lemon.

Insect Bites and Stings

A young Englishman who was visiting a neighbor in Belize was fascinated by a nearby cave high in the cliffs above the Macal River.

He was so keen to see what was inside that he laboriously climbed up the rock face, then boosted himself in.

Once inside, he let out a terrified wail. He ran out and dove head first into the river. He'd been attacked by dozens of angry bees. We counted nearly fifty stings.

He began to swell, and we thought we would have to take him to the hospital when we remembered an old-time clay remedy we had heard about from an aged healer. There was clay on the river-bank, so we decided to give it a try. We mixed it with water until it formed a paste and spread it over the stings.

It worked almost instantly. After three applications in two days he was as good as new. And wiser.

Anti-Itch Salve This halts the itching caused by mosquito, ant, and other bug bites. It also prevents infection, especially in children, who tend to scratch bites with dirty fingernails.

Put one cup each of mari-gold flowers, motherwort leaves, and basil leaves (two table-spoons each if using dried) in a glass baking dish, cover with enough olive oil to cover plants, and heat overnight in a 150-degree oven.

QUICK RELIEF

Treating Bites and Stings

Any of the following applied to the affected area will also alleviate symptoms:

- A paste of baking soda and water
- A slice of raw potato
- Lemon juice
- A fresh aloe vera piece
- An ice pack
- Peppermint toothpaste

In the morning strain the mixture through a piece of gauze to remove all traces of plant parts. Do this twice. Measure the oil. For each cup, grate two ounces of beeswax or one white candle and add slowly to the warm oil until melted. Pour off salve into a clean, wide-mouthed jar and cool. If it doesn't set, you may need to add more beeswax.

Apply to the skin several times daily (see Resources appendix).

Insomnia

There is an adorable little plant known around the world as the sensitive plant. The Maya call it sleepy head, twelve o'clock prickle, and *xmutz* (shmoots). This plant tells you how to use it: whenever you touch it, the leaves close up and look like they are falling asleep.

There are various ways to prepare the plant as a sleep aid. Some Maya toast the leaves and stems, then reduce them to a tasteless powder by passing the mixture through a sieve. They sprinkle the powder into the last meal of the day. Others like to smoke the powdered leaves in a corn husk.

You can purchase this fun plant at most nurseries. It grows wild in warm climates.

ANCIENT WISDOM

Maya Lullaby

Maya grannies place nine 6-inch branches of the sensitive plant in a cross pattern under the pillow to aid sleep in children and adults.

Kava Kava Root One of the world's top-selling herbs for anxiety and insomnia is kava kava, also known as piper. Although harvested from the South Pacific, where it has been a part of ritual and ceremony for centuries, kava kava has very close cousins in Central America. The Maya use their piper plants, called Spanish elder, for similar purposes. Their baths of piper leaves are wonderful sleep inducers.

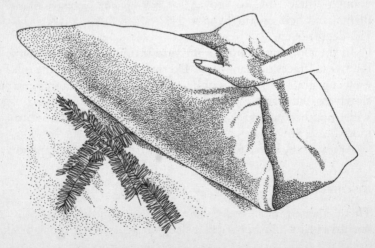

Intestinal Parasites

I've lived in the Central American tropics for thirty years and have rarely had problems with intestinal parasites once I learned how to protect myself from the invisible invaders. Prevention is the best strategy.

FROM THE KITCHEN
Papaya Seeds

An old Aztec lady taught me to eat papaya seeds to prevent intestinal parasites. "Every time you open a papaya, eat a teaspoonful of the raw seeds," she advised. They have a distinctively spicy, peppery flavor. The papain in the seeds is a protein-digesting enzyme that breaks down the cell walls of the parasites. For those who already have intestinal parasites, she suggested eating one cup of boiled, green papaya for ten days as a vegetable.

Papaya seeds can be dried and powdered in the coffee grinder. Mix a tablespoon in half a cup of water once a day before meals for ten days. Or add the papaya seed powder to salad dressings. Be sure to get your stool rechecked after the ten-day course.

I owe my good fortune to careful hygiene and two precious plants—our dear jackass bitters and raw garlic. I never travel without them. I keep a mixture of jackass bitters soaked in red wine for ten days on the kitchen counter and give a spoonful to everyone daily. We also eat raw garlic every day.

Epazote Epazote is the most respected historical treatment for parasites. To prepare, mix a teaspoon of fresh epazote juice in a quarter-cup of milk. Drink it before breakfast for nine

ANCIENT WISDOM
Wait for a New Moon

Maya custom is to start the anti-parasite treatment on the new-moon phase, that is, when there is no moon in the sky. The Maya believe that this is the time when the parasites are at their most vulnerable.

days. On the tenth day take a tablespoon of castor oil with half a glass of orange juice. Watch to see what passes.

Liver Ailments

I lived in San Francisco during the summer of love in 1968. I had the time of my life, *and* my liver suffered for it. The experience left me with a lifetime admiration for this organ.

The liver—which cleans blood by filtering it—is in need of occasional housecleaning. The Maya have some of the best liver cleansers that I know.

If you have hepatitis or a weak liver, you should see a health practitioner. Once you do, here are some helpful suggestions.

ANCIENT WISDOM
Anger and the Liver

The Maya consider the liver the seat of anger. Shamans or h'mens like Don Elijio help people release their emotions, thus lifting some of the burden off the liver.

Lemon and Water Lemon and water as a daily regime taken before breakfast is a long-respected liver cleanser. Juice one lemon and mix in a glass of tepid water. Lemon alkalinizes the blood, making for a healthy body.

Parsley Eat lots of fresh parsley. If you're lucky enough to be a gardener and have it around, you can make vegetable parsley juice daily and enjoy a glass of this before dinner. To prepare, blend half a cup of parsley leaves, half a beet, and a carrot. Strain and enjoy.

Radish Leaves You are throwing away the most nutritious part of the radish when you toss out their mineral and vitamin-rich dark green leaves. Add a few of the radish leaves to the salad. You will hardly notice them. Radish leaves can also be added to soups and sautés.

Onions Maya healers say eating lots of onions, both cooked and raw, keeps the liver healthy, clean, and working well.

Poison Ivy

Wherever poison ivy grows, its antidote, jewelweed, grows not far away. I've seen the two growing together outside New York City and in meadows and yards all over America.

Jewelweed is a wild impatients with a pale orange flower. Here's how you use it to treat the swelling, pain, and itching of poison ivy.

Mash fresh jewelweed and apply it directly to the affected area. Or place the crushed jewelweed on a piece of cotton or gauze and lay it directly over the skin. Bind it with a cloth. Jewelweed also can help prevent the poison rash if you rub some of its juice on your hands and arms ahead of time.

QUICK RELIEF

Baking Soda

Mix one tablespoon of baking soda with enough water to form a paste and apply it every hour. Peppermint toothpaste works well too.

Jewelweed Salve To prepare, collect two entire plants of jewelweed (one large one will do), then wash and remove dirt from the roots. Blend thoroughly with enough olive oil to make the mixture about the consistency of pesto. Heat the mixture overnight in a 150-degree oven.

While the mixture is still warm, strain it through cheesecloth and add six ounces of grated beeswax or one white candle. Stir until smooth and well blended. Bottle in clean wide-mouthed glass containers and store away for summertime use. This salve has a shelf life of about eighteen months and lasts longer if refrigerated. Be sure to date and label the jar.

Gumbo-limbo Salve Gumbo-limbo trees grow in most southern and western states. The red, shaggy bark is extremely effective against poison ivy and poisonwood. We make a healing salve from the gumbo-limbo bark by steeping two cups of gumbo-limbo bark and two cups of vegetable shortening in the oven overnight at 150 degrees, then straining and bottling it in the morning. If you don't want to make this salve yourself, order some "Jungle Salve" (see the Resources appendix).

Psoriasis and Eczema

People with eczema suffer from itching and painful scaly lesions. Those with psoriasis have reddish patches covered with silver scales and a thickening of the skin surface. Psoriasis can be chronic and often responds only temporarily to cortisone treatment.

I group eczema and psoriasis together here because conventional wisdom has it that both conditions are caused by an overload of toxins in the bloodstream.

The Maya keep their blood clean by eating a lot of juicy fruits such as papaya, pineapples, oranges, melons, and watermelons and by drinking gumbo-limbo and wild yam tea and plenty of water.

Gumbo-limbo and Wild Yam Tea   Boil a quarter-cup of dried gumbo-limbo bark and a quarter-cup of dried wild yam in one quart of water for twenty minutes. Steep for twenty minutes. Strain. Sip the tea all day.

Natural Pharmacist Dan Wagner's Salve   Every year a group of pharmacy students from Duquesne University comes to Ix Chel Farm for a "Pharmacy from the Rainforest" course. Their group leader, and the founder of this unique program, is the natural pharmacist Dan Wagner.

Wagner was intrigued with the quick action of our gumbo-limbo salve on mosquito bites, rashes, and poisonwood. He took a few jars home and tried the salve on psoriasis and eczema. He combined the salve with aloe vera, vitamin E, and a tiny amount of cortisone. It works wonders and is a longer-lasting cure than cortisone alone (see the Resources appendix for more information).

Ringworm

While working on this book at home in Belize, I developed a red, round, weepy patch of skin on my arm. Within the day it was clear that a viral infection known as ringworm had settled in.

Pumpkin Vine Leaves   One of the Maya's favorite ringworm remedies is a combination of the juice of one fresh lemon (lime works too), a pinch of salt, and a leaf of the pumpkin vine.

To prepare, pick a leaf from a mature vine growing in full sunlight. Blend with the juice and salt, adding more juice until the concoction is the consistency of paste.

Rub the paste on the ringworm several times daily or place on a gauze pad that you tape over the skin and change three times daily.

When the leaves of the pumpkin vine are not available, Maya women make a paste with crushed garlic, castor oil, and a pinch of salt.

Basil   The Maya also use fresh basil leaves to treat ringworm. Crush the leaves with salt and lay on as a poultice. Secure in place with a strip of cotton cloth. Keep this on overnight, but let the ringworm air during the day.

Flowers of Sulfur and Aloe   *Tinea alba* is a variety of ringworm that leaves white patches on the body. This is a very stubborn condition, but I've seen great results with the following treatment.

We always keep some flowers of sulfur powder on hand. Sulfur powder is available at almost any pharmacy without prescription. I combine the sulfur with the juice of an aloe vera plant and a few drops of vitamin E. I mash it up with my fingers and apply it directly to the white patch. Keep the area clean with soap and water. Apply at least three times daily, and you will get results.

Flowers of sulfur need to be treated with caution and respect. Be careful not to get the powder into open sores, eyes, or mucus membranes. Do not breathe in sulfur dust. Sulfur powder becomes sulfuric acid when it comes in contact with mucus membranes. Discontinue at first signs of redness or rawness of the skin.

Sore Throat

A sore throat usually means that your immune system is gearing up for a battle against an infection or virus. Here are a few remedies to help alleviate the discomfort.

Tomato Juice Cocktail   The tomato, one of the gifts of the New World to the Old, boasts many medicinal qualities.

To prepare a cocktail, blend eight ounces of tomato juice (you could also use one or two fresh garden tomatoes), the juice of one

ANCIENT WISDOM

Sore Throat Pressure Point

Don Elijio used to pinch *hard* the fleshy skin between the thumb and forefinger (the large intestine four point). His patients would squirm and struggle to get away, but he held them fast. Don Elijio believed that pinching this pressure point pushed out congested blood and reduced the swelling.

lemon, and two or three cloves of garlic for a few minutes. Drink the cocktail cooler than room temperature. Sip slowly and allow the juice to flow over the back of your throat. Add ice for a more soothing effect. This remedy brings quick relief. Repeat throughout the day.

Stomach Complaints

Thanks to years of belly dancing and a good clean diet I almost never have any stomach problems. But lots of other people do. Most of Don Elijio's patients came to his clinic complaining of gastritis. He blamed this on "cold machines"—his term for refrigerators and freezers. He didn't approve of factory-made food either.

Among the most useful treatments I learned in my ten-year apprenticeship with Don Elijio were those for stomach trouble, what the Maya call *ciro* (seero), which can include the following symptoms:

Feeling full after eating only a little bit of food
Indigestion
Nausea
Flatulence
Heartburn
Weakness of the legs
Constipation
Diarrhea
Headache
Weight loss or weight gain

The Maya believe that these symptoms are primarily caused by drinking a cold beverage while eating hot food. Maya reasoning is that the sudden cold causes the expanded, warm muscles of the stomach to go into spasm, thereby causing lack of appetite, indigestion, and pain. I think they're on to something. Many people who suffer from stomach complaints do drink a lot of cold drinks with meals and like to chew on ice.

There is another characteristic that people who suffer from chronic gastritis have in common. The area between the rib cage and the stomach is as hard as a rock and hurts when pressure is applied. This painful knot is an emotional block that has the stomach muscles tied up in spasms and is exacerbated by cold drinks. The stomach area is the seat of anxiety, fear, and worry.

Maya healers always include a deep, penetrating stomach massage with their treatment for ciro (see part 3, "Bodywork"). It also helps to lay a hot water bottle or a heating pad set on low over your stomach at bedtime for half an hour. Do this every night for a week and then twice a week after that.

Don Elijio's Anti-Ciro Remedy
Medicinal plants are part of every Maya treatment for stomach problems. These are used to relax the stomach muscles and improve digestion and circulation to the digestive organs. I know of no better formula than Don Elijio's own, made of three jungle vines known as guinweo, man vine, and guaco. The remedy gently cleans the bowels and eases

QUICK RELIEF FOR NAUSEA

Orange
When you cannot keep down any liquids, calm your stomach spasms by sniffing a crushed fresh orange leaf or rind. For nausea with indigestion, make an orange rind or leaf tea.

Peppermint Tea
Peppermint tea is a time-honored home remedy for nausea. Boil one tablespoon of dried peppermint leaves or half a cup of fresh peppermint leaves and stems in one cup of water for five minutes. Steep for fifteen minutes, then slowly drink the tea warm and unsweetened. Inhale the aroma while drinking.

Peppermint Quick Fix
The quickest way to get rid of nausea is to pinch off a few leaves of peppermint, wash them, and pop them into your mouth. Chew and swallow.

heartburn and gas. He called this formula *sacca todo,* or "pull out everything." I call it "Belly Be Good" (see the Resources appendix).

Peppermint for Indigestion If indigestion hits at home, I eat several leaves of fresh peppermint. When I am traveling, I've adapted this old custom to modern times. I swallow half a teaspoon of all-natural peppermint or fennel toothpaste. Sometimes I have to do this twice.

FROM THE KITCHEN
A Case of Bad Gas

Culinary spices found their way into our food because they are tasty digestive aids that prevent spoiling and calm stomach upsets.

Once a dear friend called me at midnight in the middle of a Chicago blizzard. "Rosita!" she said frantically. "My dad hasn't slept for two nights because of terrible gas pains in his belly. Is there anything you can suggest? We're desperate to help him."

"What spices do you have in your kitchen cabinet that are less than a year old?" I asked.

"Oregano, rosemary, thyme, basil, and sage," she replied.

"All right, boil a heaping tablespoonful of any three of them in two cups of water for ten minutes. Let it sit for ten minutes. Strain it and give it to your dad piping hot."

She called back within the hour, sounding less frantic.

"My dad is sound asleep. The stomach cramps stopped almost immediately, and within a half-hour he was sleeping like a baby. Who would have imagined such a simple remedy could work so well and quickly?"

Styes

Styes are contagious bacterial infections of the eyelids that cause pain, swelling, and a little red pimple. Sties are common in school-age children. Here's what I was taught to do by the traditional healers.

Chamomile When my daughter was in sixth grade, she came home with her first sty. I prepared the following strong brew.

Boil three tablespoons (or three tea bags) of chamomile flowers in one and a half cups of water for five minutes. Steep for ten minutes. If using the flowers, strain through cheesecloth. Be sure to remove *all* traces of plant parts.

I always keep a little eye-wash cup on hand. It looks a bit like a holder for a boiled egg. Place a teaspoon of the tea in the cup and place it over the eye. Let the tea bathe the eye and lid. Repeat three times.

By the way, I use this same remedy on my two Doberman pinschers when they get eye infections, although they are harder to treat than a child.

ANCIENT WISDOM

Foods to Avoid

Some good, sensible advice from the Maya: whenever an infection is present, avoid bananas, avocados, peanuts, milk, cheese, and sugar. These foods delay healing and encourage the formation of pus.

If the sty doesn't start to improve in thirty-six hours, add raw garlic to the diet. Those who can't eat raw garlic—including children—can be given two garlic oil capsules every six hours until the sty is better.

Swelling

When my husband, Greg, and I went to Madrid, we visited Alex, a young man who had interned on our farm the year before. A few months before we arrived, Alex's father had fallen and hurt his leg. Drawing on what he had learned in Belize, Alex treated his Dad's painfully swollen calf.

"It was so amazing!" his dad explained. "My son went to the kitchen cabinet and said, 'I remember seeing Rosita do this.'"

Alex had boiled a strong pot of sage tea and soaked strips of cotton cloth in it. When the cloths cooled to room temperature, he wrapped them around his father's calf.

"I went to sleep that night with my foot resting on a pillow wrapped up like a mummy and smelling like soup," Alex's father went on. "By the next day my leg swelling was way down—about 90 percent improved. It was incredible!"

This is an easy remedy to try at home.

Sage Boil one cup of fresh sage (or two tablespoons of dried sage) in one quart of water for ten minutes. Steep until cool. If swelling isn't reduced within twenty-four hours, see a doctor.

Aloe Some healers break open aloe and rub the gel on the swelling. Others heat the aloe first. The American herbal guru Jim Duke says in his book *Green Pharmacy* that aloe contains an enzyme that decreases swelling and pain.

Toothaches

When I was a kid, my Assyrian auntie Emma Eshoo used to give us cloves to chew on when we had a toothache. Later it came as no surprise that Maya healers often use cloves for the same purpose. The Maya like allspice even better.

Allspice tastes a lot like cloves because the two spices share some of the same chemicals. The chemical eugenol, for example, gives both spices their flavor and acts quickly, but temporarily, on painful teeth and gums.

FROM THE KITCHEN

Allspice Berry for Toothaches

Break up a few whole allspice berries by chewing and place the crushed seed on the gum near the tooth that hurts. The allspice does nothing for your cavity but will alleviate the pain until you can get help.

Yarrow If you're out in the woods on a hike when a toothache strikes, look for feathery yarrow leaves. Chomp down on one or two and place the mash against the gum where the tooth hurts. I've done this for myself and friends many a time with amazingly quick results.

Ulcers

Don Elijio always prescribed his favorite plant, skunk root, for ulcers of the digestive tract with excellent results.

I use the skunk root whenever patients tell me that everything else they have tried has failed. I cannot tell you why it works so well on stubborn cases, but my guess would be that it creates an unfavorable environment for the bacteria now suspected to cause ulcers. Skunk root also has another benefit for the high-strung people who tend to develop ulcers: the Maya use it to treat the spiritual and emotional ailments that may underlie the condition. Skunk root is not easily available in the northern climes, but it can be ordered, along with instructions for proper use (see the Resources appendix).

Here are a few Maya home remedies that also work.

Raw Cabbage Juice   A good old-fashioned universal remedy for ulcers is fresh, raw cabbage juice. Half a head of cabbage juiced makes about two cups. Drink one cup twice daily between meals. Raw cabbage can also be eaten throughout the day if chewed well and slowly.

Honey   Some Maya healers recommend one tablespoon of honey at bedtime every day for at least two weeks. Honey is used in many countries around the world for the same purpose. Honey builds up the lining of the stomach and destroys bacteria. You need raw, uncooked honey to get the benefits. Ask for it at your health food store.

Plantains   When green, plantain, the large bananalike fruit available in grocery stores, has an enzyme that increases the amount of healing mucus in the stomach lining.

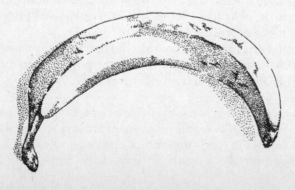

To prepare, peel the skin from two green plantains. Chop and boil in enough water to cover until the plantain is soft. This should take about fifteen minutes. Add three tablespoons of honey and mash with a fork. Eat half a cup before meals for several days.

Warts

Warts are commonly found on the feet, hands, arms, and face. They are viral in origin and look like raised brownish growths on the skin. In Maya they are known as *ax* (awsh). The following treatments are easy and efficient.

Green Papaya The classic Maya treatment for warts is the white milky sap that runs from the green papaya. Papain, a protein digestive enzyme in papaya, is the therapeutic agent. Place the sap on a gauze and put it over the wart.

If you happen to live where papayas grow, lucky you. Go to the tree and poke a green papaya with your fingernail. Collect the white sap onto a cotton swab. Rub it on the wart a few times each day.

If you don't live near a papaya tree, go to the grocery store. Green papayas are available throughout the United States and Europe. Although the papayas in the store have little milky sap, the green skin has enough papain in it to do the job.

Score it lightly on the inside and the outside. Place it over the wart and wrap it with a piece of cloth or gauze bandage. Change the dressing once a day.

Apply the skin or milky sap for ten days. Expect a temporary burning sensation when the papain begins to digest the wart. The burning sensation doesn't last long and is harmless to healthy skin. If you have what looks like a more serious reaction—a blister or a rash—discontinue the treatment.

The digestive enzyme papain can also be purchased in capsule or powder form at a health food store. Mix the powder into a paste with castor oil. Apply to warts several times daily.

Garlic If a green papaya is not available or you experience a reaction to papaya, try garlic. Garlic oil capsules are easy to use and can be found in any health food store. Break open a capsule and rub the oil vigorously over the wart three times daily. Some folks have good results with raw, crushed garlic. Apply it several times daily as a poultice. Place in a strip of gauze bandage and change twice daily. The only problem is the odor.

Plantar Warts Plantar warts occur on the bottom of the feet and make it hard to walk or stand without pain. Make a paste out of one tablespoon of castor oil and one teaspoon of baking soda and apply to the plantar wart. Keep in place with a strip of clean cotton. Change every evening and morning. The time this treatment takes to work depends on the size of the wart. Expect that it will take at least ten days.

Wrinkles

Maya people are fortunate to have smooth copper-colored complexions that don't wrinkle much until around age seventy. Until then, they seem to maintain an almost ageless status. Here are some of their wrinkle prevention therapies.

Avocado Cream Mash ripe avocados with a fork and apply to the face, neck, and hands. Leave on for twenty minutes. Wash off with clear water and repeat once or twice weekly.

Hibiscus and Rose Lotion The red and pink flowering hibiscus is highly medicinal and contains lotionlike mucilage that is beneficial to the skin. Red roses are mildly astringent and nourishing.

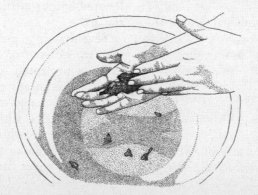

To prepare, mash three open red or pink hibiscus (or hollyhock) flowers and one red rose in a basin containing a cup of water. Rub the flowers back and forth between your hands for five minutes. Add more water if needed. Strain through a cheesecloth. Apply to the face, neck, and hands two or three times daily. Bottle in a clean jar. This lotion will last a few months if refrigerated.

Physical Ailments of Women

A constant stream of women came to see Don Elijio with menstrual and uterine problems. Gaggles of six or more would arrive in a taxi or climb down off the back of a pickup truck, giggling as if they were on their way to a party. The group social activity was a visit to the old Maya healer for uterine balancing sessions.

The Maya believe that female problems usually have one source: a uterus that has dropped from its proper position in the pelvis. This may sound odd to modern ears since the effects of a dropped uterus are almost completely ignored by our medical practitioners.

Seventy-five percent of women suffer from what is called a prolapsed, or tipped, uterus. This means that many women are being treated for female troubles without ever having the underlying cause addressed. As a result, Maya women under the care of traditional healers often receive better care than women under conventional medical care.

Xeno-Estrogen

If you want to control hormonal blues of any kind, watch out for xeno-estrogens or estrogens from foreign sources. Eat only organic meats, dairy products, and chickens that are grown without the hormones that make them abnormally fat. Xeno-estrogens play havoc with a woman's body by upsetting the delicate feedback system between the ovaries, the uterine lining, and the hypothalamus in the brain—thus the uncharacteristic extremes of highs and lows that cause us to feel way off balance. Include a lot of soy products in your diet. Soy contains phyto-estrogens, which block receptor sites for damaging xeno-estrogens.

"The uterus is a woman's center, and if it is not in good position and condition, nothing in her life will be right," Don Elijio used to declare. "The periods will be late, early, and painful."

The uterus is hung like a hammock across the pelvis. The ligaments that hold it have a tendency to overstretch, thus allowing the uterus to sag and fall into various improper positions. Obviously, flexible ligaments are essential for pregnancy and childbirth.

Causes of a prolapsed uterus include falls that injure the sacrum, poor professional care during pregnancy and childbirth, running on concrete surfaces, high-impact dancing and sports, surgical errors, and heavy lifting.

Included on the following pages are a wide range of Maya home remedies for women. However, the foundation of women's health is the placement of the uterus. Turn to part 3, "Bodywork," for more information about the prolapsed uterus and step-by-step instructions for the self-help centering massage.

Eating a good diet and exercising are also important components of women's health. Here are a few general tips.

Increase your water intake to eight glasses daily.

Avoid cold drinks and foods before and during your period. Drink only warm or room-temperature liquids at that time.

Eliminate dairy products (except natural yogurt) and white flour from your diet.

Also eat less meat and sugar.

Don't drink more than an occasional cup of coffee.

Get up, girl, and move! There is no excuse not to get in at least twenty minutes a day of walking, stretching, yoga, or working out with weights. Belly dancing is the primo exercise for female troubles because it was originally intended to increase female pelvic health and ensure fertility.

Amenorrhea

Amenorrhea, or lack of menstruation, has many possible causes. Low body fat can be a factor, especially in adolescent girls, dancers, thin women, and women who work out excessively. Exhaustion, malnutrition, and stress play a role. Lack of menstruation can also be due to an imbalance between estrogen and progesterone.

Sometimes women who have recently switched to a vegetarian diet experience temporary cessation of menstruation.

The main Maya treatment for amenorrhea is the abdominal massage (see part 3, "Bodywork"), which increases blood circulation to and from the uterus and ovaries. Healers prescribe the vaginal steam bath twice a week (see below), and a purge to clean out the bowels is also given (see the purges described under "Constipation" in the section on general ailments). Last but not least, herbal teas are prescribed. Women who may be pregnant should avoid all of these treatments.

Last year while lecturing in Turin, Italy, I treated a twenty-six-year-old woman who had not had a period in more than a year. I found that her uterus had slipped down and was leaning far to the left.

I performed a five-minute Maya abdominal massage, then taught her how to do the massage for herself. I told her to drink oregano tea for three days.

ANCIENT WISDOM
The Vaginal Steam Bath

Vaginal steam baths are an old, respected treatment for women used by Maya midwives and healers. *Bajos* (ba-hoes), as they are called in Spanish, are a common and effective treatment for many female complaints, especially those of a serious or chronic nature. Vaginal steam baths are also good preventive care. They are mentioned many times in this section of the book.

Some of the most commonly used plants for the vaginal steam bath are oregano, basil, marigold, and rosemary. If you have these in your garden, pick a double handful of fresh leaves and stems—about a quart jar loosely filled. Use one herb or any combination. If using dried herbs, you need one cup of herbs.

Boil in a gallon of water for ten minutes and steep for five minutes. Remove the pot from the stove and place it under a chair with open slits—a cane, wood, or plastic yard chair will work.

The woman removes her clothes from the waist down, including underwear. She sits on the chair over the steaming herbs, and is then covered with a blanket from the waist down. This keeps the steam contained under the blanket. Be sure she feels comfortable with the steam temperature and is not exposed to cold drafts. Wrap her upper body in a dry, warm blanket.

Exactly three days later she called. "Che buono" (How great), she exclaimed. Her period had arrived. She has had no further problems with her cycle.

Herbal Teas Here's how to make teas to treat amenorrhea. Boil one cup of fresh oregano, basil, or rosemary or a combination of all three (or three tablespoons of any single herb or herb combination in dried form) in three cups of water for five minutes. Steep for fifteen minutes. Drink one cup—between meals and as hot as possible—during the course of the day.

Tincture Don Elijio came up with a wonderful formula, consisting mainly of wild yam, China root, and ginger, that he called "Female Tonic." It is too complicated to make on your own (see Resources appendix).

The steam bath, which introduces a lot of healing heat into the uterus, should last twenty minutes.

Afterward have the woman lie in bed for an hour under warm covers. The steam bath may be repeated every two weeks as a treatment, and twice a year for prevention.

Other herbs useful for vaginal steam baths include burdock leaves, motherwort, Saint-John's-wort, chamomile damiana, plantain horsetail, red clover yarrow, Mexican wormseed (epazote), dandelion, yellow dock, and squaw vine.

Childbirth

Thousands of years of necessity have created a sophisticated and comprehensive Maya care plan for pregnancy, childbirth, and post-delivery care.

Maya midwives are remarkable, dedicated women with skills that have been fine-tuned by generations of use. Traditional home birth attendants and midwives play an important role because even today most Maya babies are delivered at home.

Morning Sickness Midwives view vomiting in the first trimester as a good thing and counsel their clients to be patient. They believe that vomiting is evidence that the body is cleaning itself to prepare a favorable environment for the growing fetus.

When relief of morning sickness is required, the Maya midwife recommends that the soon-to-be mom suck on the dried fruit of the tamarind tree. She sprinkles the fruit with a bit of salt. (This sour fruit is available in Spanish stores under the name "Tamarindo.")

> ## QUICK RELIEF
> ### Sniffing Nausea Away
> Place a slice of orange or lemon peel under the pregnant woman's nose. She should squeeze and sniff repeatedly.

In extreme cases warm tea made from one teaspoon of cumin seeds or cumin powder is boiled with a clove of peeled garlic for ten minutes. Steep until warm and sip slowly.

Later Pregnancy Maya midwives address most problems or complications of pregnancy by performing the abdominal massage, ensuring a full complement of blood supply and proper positioning of the uterus and fetus. Abdominal massage during pregnancy should be done only by professionals (see Resources appendix to locate practitioners).

Spotting During Pregnancy As soon as spotting begins, Maya women prepare a tea from five open and four closed red hibiscus or pink and red hollyhock flowers. They boil the nine flowers with nine leaves along with half a teaspoon of powdered cinnamon in two cups of water for ten minutes. *When the concoction has cooled,* the pregnant woman sips it slowly and continuously until she has consumed all of it. The treatment is repeated if necessary.

If hibiscus or hollyhock are not available, use nine red roses and six inches of leaf and stem. Always take these teas when cooled, never warm or hot. Be sure the flowers are insecticide-free.

Maya healers also recommend bed rest with a pillow under the hips to elevate the pelvis.

Delivery The Maya midwife will see her client monthly during pregnancy to check the uterine position and that of the baby. Breech babies are turned expertly and efficiently by swinging the woman in a hammock while the uterine massage is performed.

To ensure an easy delivery, mothers are advised to be active, walk a lot, and get lots of fresh air. Maya women also eat six pieces of raw okra *or* take half a cup of desert nopal juice once daily for ten days before their due date. The slippery, mucilaginous substance in okra and nopal makes for an easy birth and has been a part of Maya midwifery care since ancient days.

During labor midwives administer as much hot allspice tea as the woman can consume. She continuously sips on the warm tea to ease the pains and to ensure steady progress. Midwives boil three tablespoons of allspice berries or powder in one quart of water for ten minutes. They let it steep for fifteen minutes, strain it, and place it in a bedside thermos.

ANCIENT WISDOM
How to Avoid Tearing

The midwife Hortence Robinson (I call her the woman of *mil secretos,* or a thousand secrets) says that in sixty years of attending women in childbirth no woman in her care has ever required stitching for tearing during delivery. Here is her secret to prevent tearing of the perineum during delivery.

1. Rub warm olive oil on the perineum and upper thighs every half-hour throughout labor as well as in between contractions during the final stage.
2. Do not allow the woman to have her feet off the bed. The feet must be planted firmly on the surface of the bed, never held up in midair.

If labor seems too slow or begins to recede, midwives prescribe hot ginger tea and if necessary will soak a towel in the hot tea and place it over the abdomen.

FROM THE KITCHEN

Excessive Bleeding

For excessive bleeding after delivery, the Maya midwife gives cool teas of either red hibiscus or roses mixed with cinnamon. I have watched Miss Hortence use this successfully many times.

In 1993 I was invited to Guatemala to work with an independent group of American nurses who were running a clinic for remote villagers along the Rio Dulce River. They asked me to share with them how they could incorporate safe, reliable, and easily available home remedies into their daily clinic practice.

One day a father and son came into the clinic carrying a hammock. In the hammock was an emaciated Maya woman who was too weak to stand or sit up. Her complexion was muddy gray, and her eyes would not focus.

Three months before, the husband reported, the woman had miscarried her eleventh child. She had been bleeding vaginally ever since.

I remembered Miss Hortence's great success with the hibiscus and cinnamon tea and asked the nurses for permission to treat her. They agreed, and I set to work.

I found the red hibiscus growing directly outside the clinic door, then went to the kitchen for some cinnamon. I prepared the tea, cooled it, and gave her half-cup doses every fifteen minutes.

When she got up to urinate, there was still some blood present. After an hour there was less, and finally after two hours, there was none. The bleeding had finally stopped.

Her husband fell to his knees and cried, saying, "Senora! My poor wife has lain in her sick bed for three months, and all the time the red hibiscus was at her window and we didn't know it could help her."

Postdelivery The midwife visits the mother's home for nine days following delivery to make sure that both mother and child are doing well. Some Maya midwives also prepare meals, wash clothing, care for older children, and clean house for nine days—thus the term "mid-wife."

The presence of the midwife during these early days after delivery is considered vitally important. It prevents the mother from working too hard or rising from her bed too soon. Returning to normal domestic activity too soon is one of the major causes of the prolapsed uterus.

A vaginal steam bath and uterine massage are given on the third day to ensure complete cleansing of the uterus, prevent infection, and guide the uterus back to its proper position.

Dysmenorrhea

Painful periods is such a common complaint that some women have come to believe that such pain is normal. This isn't true. A normal period should be either painless or involve, at most, half an hour of cramping. Any more than that is too much.

Most of the time dysmenorrhea is caused by the prolapsed uterus and, in some cases, underlying emotional issues. The Maya also consider a woman with menstrual cramps to be suffering from a "cold" disease. Cold diseases are characterized by cramping and muscle tightness.

Maya healers believe that the period is painful because the prolapsed uterus is not able to flush itself out completely from month to month. The menstrual blood that remains behind hardens and thickens. The next period is painful because the body uses more

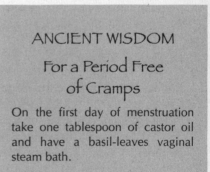

ANCIENT WISDOM

For a Period Free
of Cramps

On the first day of menstruation take one tablespoon of castor oil and have a basil-leaves vaginal steam bath.

force to try to eliminate this encrusted material. The body uses more and more force with each cycle.

Treatment includes the external uterine massage (see part 3, "Bodywork," for instructions), herbs, and, in stubborn cases, a vaginal steam bath between periods. The uterine massage returns the uterus to its proper position and strengthens the ligaments. Teas taken for ten days before the onset of menses help flush out the remaining material from the uterus.

Don't be afraid of what flows out. It's often a very dark brown, thick fluid. It may take three to five periods before all of the material is loosened from the uterine membrane.

Red Hibiscus Flowers A tea made of red hibiscus flowers has long been the favorite Maya treatment for painful periods. Nine flowers are eaten for painful menses and excessive menstruation with cramping. Hibiscus is in the okra family, so if you can't find them, eat a handful of raw okra or a serving of cooked okra.

Hot Ginger Tea Grate one tablespoon of fresh ginger. Boil in one and a half cups of water for ten minutes. Steep for ten minutes and take as hot as possible.

Hot Basil, Rosemary, or Oregano Tea Boil a cup of fresh herbs (or three teaspoons of dried herbs) in three cups of water for five minutes. Steep for ten minutes. Drink as hot as possible.

If you have tried all of these herbal treatments and performed the uterine massage on yourself and you still have painful periods, you are a candidate for the Maya vaginal steam bath (see pages 92–93).

Endometriosis

Endometriosis is a painful condition that occurs when the uterine tissues are forced out of the uterus and into the fallopian tubes by intense cramping during menstruation. The errant bits of uterine lining can attach themselves anywhere in the body. A healthy immune system should destroy this renegade tissue. When the immune system is too weak to react, the tissue begins to grow. It behaves just like uterine cells and menstruates every month.

Don Elijio believed that endometriosis is caused by the prolapsed uterus (see part 3, "Bodywork," for more details). After the uterus has been centered, take the following herbal preparations.

Rue Tea Maya healers recommend taking rue three times daily for ten days prior to menstruation. This is followed up by a tablespoon of castor oil on the first day of menstruation.

Mash nine small branches (two to three inches in length with leaves) into one and a half cups of warm water. Strain and drink one half-cup before meals three times daily. If using dried rue, steep a large tablespoon in one and a half cups of hot water for twenty minutes.

Motherwort Tea If rue isn't available, try motherwort, a common wild herb found all over the Americas and Europe. It can also be purchased in dried form in health food stores.

Boil two 12-inch branches with leaves and stems in three cups of water for ten minutes and steep for twenty minutes. Drink in half-cup doses three times daily for ten days before menstruation.

Endometritis

Endometritis is inflammation of the lining of the uterus—the endometrium. From the Maya perspective, it is caused by the pro lapsed uterus. When not in its proper place, the uterus is unable to clean itself well, and inflammation and infection can result.

Symptoms include pelvic pain with menstruation, burning, bleeding between cycles, infertility, chronic miscarriages, painful intercourse, vaginal discharge, and backache.

Endometritis does not get better overnight. See part 3, "Body-work," for instruction on performing the external uterine massage. Here are some herbs that also help.

Red Hibiscus Tea A tea of red hibiscus or mallow flowers can soothe the inflammation and pain. Boil nine open flowers and nine leaves in three cups of water for ten minutes. Drink at room temperature in three doses or sip throughout the day.

Fibroids

Fibroids have become distressingly common among modern women all over the world. They are benign growths in the uterus that can grow to a large size and cause pain, backache, headaches, excessive bleeding, and a host of other female problems.

The flurry of fibroids may be traceable to a diet that consists of hormone-raised meat, dairy products, sugar, processed food, and caffeine. Another cause may be artificial estrogen, like the estrogen found in birth control pills.

How Estrogen Works

Estrogen stimulates cells to grow. Women need it to build up the lining of the uterus in preparation for menstruation and to increase the capacity of our breasts to hold mother's milk for babies. During and after menopause, estrogen adds fat to our bodies where it can be stored for use throughout the rest of life.

When we consume estrogens from outside our bodies, it creates anarchy in the cells. Estrogen must proliferate! It is driven by a need to grow. An unhealthy uterus in a body flooded with artificial estrogen is very likely to produce fibroids and other growths.

Uterine fibroids are not easy to treat, and results take time. Maya healers suggest uterine massage, the vaginal steam baths, and herbs. The herbs need to be both cleansing and astringent in order to shrink the fibroids and then stimulate the uterine lining to slough off the shrunken tissue. Miss Hortence dispensed a complex special formula that is very difficult to make (see Resources appendix).

Infertility

As Maya midwives know, there is no simple answer or cause for infertility. It can be due to environmental factors, stress, anxiety, emotional inability to accept becoming a parent, aversion to pregnancy and weight gain, scarred uterine lining, hormonal imbalance, or blocked fallopian tubes. In rare cases the woman's own body destroys the sperm. The first thing a Maya healer does is look for signs of a prolapsed uterus with an unhealthy lining.

A visitor to Belize from the United States came to Ix Chel Farm to consult with me about her lifetime problems with menstruation and then infertility. Marie was forty-two years old and had delayed family life in favor of a journalism career. Recently married, she was now in a rush to get pregnant.

Her husband's sperm had been tested and was normal and motile. Her history showed that she had had painful periods most of her life. "I feel a heavy bearing down, like something is going to fall out of me, before my period starts," she explained.

She also had premenstrual syndrome: dark, thick blood at the beginning and the end of menstruation, lower back ache and headaches with her period, and painful sex.

Marie had a prolapsed uterus with classic symptoms. As we talked, she revealed that as an equestrienne in college she had suffered several severe falls. She was now a runner and, because she lived in Chicago, ran on hard surfaces.

Gentle external massage in the first treatment was somewhat painful for Marie. I showed her husband how to do the massage for her, cautioning him not to press too deeply.

Because they were guests at a nearby jungle resort for the next two weeks, I was able to see Marie three more times. By the second visit her uterus had begun to correct itself. I fixed her a vaginal steam bath as well.

By the time she left for home her period had started. She was amazed at the amount of dark, thick, foul-smelling fluids she passed. "Some of it looked like chunks of flesh," she exclaimed.

Marie e-mailed me several times when she got back to the States. She was pregnant within three months, although she miscarried in the first trimester. Soon after she conceived again. That time she delivered a healthy eight-pound baby boy.

Herbs A woman experiencing infertility needs a good uterine cleanser until her normal menstrual flow becomes pink and watery. There are several good women's formulas on the market these days, and they are readily available from health food stores. I like those that contain wild yam along with other herbs. I can also recommend motherwort—an excellent herb for women's ailments. The Maya use fresh motherwort because they love bitter teas. "The bitterer the better," goes the expression. You may prefer capsules or tincture from the health food store. Follow the instructions on the label for ten days before your period three cycles in a row. While you are taking motherwort, don't try to get pregnant.

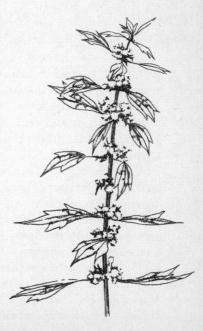

Menopause

Menopause, the cessation or pause of the monthly cycle (in Greek the word for month is *mens*), is a gradual transition from the child-bearing to the crone years. It can occur anywhere from age thirty-five to age fifty, depending on your genes.

Menopause should be a time of joy, wisdom-sharing, and release from the responsibilities of the childbearing years. Historically, menopausal women were the wise women who gave good counsel based on their decades of experience. It is only recently that menopause has begun to be dreaded as difficult.

Maya women too have begun to suffer from difficult menopause. Several Maya elders I know have told me that until the 1960s difficult menopause was almost unknown among Maya women. What happened? They blame new perceptions about *el cambio*, in part, on processed, bottled, boxed, treated, sprayed, and chemically pro-duced artificial foods. At one time women ate only their own organically homegrown corn, beans, pumpkins, chilis, greens, seasonal fruits, and vegetables. Other factors are the extra emo-tional burdens of modern life and the message that being old is undesirable.

When menopause occurs, a woman's hormonal balance changes, making her feel out of sorts. Signs may be weight gain, dry vagina, mood swings, dry skin that wrinkles more easily, hot flashes, mem-ory loss, tearfulness, emotional swings, and insomnia. Or there may be none of the above. Some of these signs may occur up to ten years before menopause.

Healthy women with a well-positioned uterus and a natural diet that includes lots of calcium and whole foods usually have an easier time with menopause.

Several herbs will ease the transition.

FROM THE KITCHEN
Calcium Foods for Menopause

Almonds, sesame, and sunflower seeds
Amaranth, collard, and kale greens
Kelp, seaweeds, and parsley
Soybeans and soy products
Tahini

Rosy Periwinkle Tea Maya women make a tea from the common rosy periwinkle that grows in backyards everywhere. This is the same plant that gave us vincristine and vinblastine for treatment of childhood leukemia and Hodgkin's disease.

To prepare, take two branches about twelve inches in length with stems, leaves, and pink flowers. Boil in three cups of water for two minutes. Steep for fifteen minutes, then strain. Drink one cup before each meal three times daily. Follow this regime only one week out of every month.

Mexican Wild Yam Tea This common remedy for difficult menopause helps to alleviate bothersome mood swings, insomnia, hot flashes, and memory loss. Wild yam is considered by herbalists a "hormone balancer." The wild yam has steroidal compounds that help regulate the normal ebb and flow of female hormones.

Boil a small handful of dried roots in three cups of water for fifteen minutes. Steep for twenty minutes and take three cups daily before each meal, or sip slowly throughout the day.

Rosemary Tea Another favorite home remedy (look under "Premenstrual Syndrome" for preparation instructions), rosemary is one of those blessed plants that contains phyto-estrogens. Basil tea works also.

Female Tonic Don Elijio prescribed a female tonic that includes wild yam, China root, and ginger (see the Resources appendix).

Depression Tea For depression during menopause Maya women drink rosemary tea. To prepare, boil one fresh twelve-inch branch of rosemary or one tablespoon of dried rosemary in two cups of water for five minutes. Steep for ten minutes and drink warm in between meals.

Depression Bath A soothing herbal bath is another effective treatment for menopausal depression. You need three branches each of rosemary, basil, and marigold about twelve inches in length. Squeeze into a large pot of water until leaves and flowers are well crushed.

If it is summer, let the mixture sit in the sun. When the water is warm, carry the pot into your bathroom. Using a bowl, pour the herbal water over your body. Let the herbal water air-dry on your skin, out in the sunshine if possible.

If it is not summertime and fresh plants are not available, use half a cup each of dried rosemary, basil, and marigold. Dried marigold is impossible to buy, so if you want to use it, plan ahead and dry your own. Otherwise, rosemary and basil will do fine.

Boil the herbs in a gallon of water for twenty minutes. Steep for twenty more minutes. Pour into your bathtub and soak in this bath for half an hour. Light incense or a candle, and relax.

Menstrual Irregularity

The normal menstrual cycle varies from twenty-one to forty-five days. The cycle that has no pattern or comes and goes at random is irregular. Irregular cycles are most common in teenagers, who eventually become more regular with the passing of years.

The ebb and flow of the female cycle is intricate and fascinating. Menstruation is controlled by minute amounts of the hormones estriol, estrone, and estradiol. These together are what we think of as estrogen. Progesterone and other hormones also play a role.

The balance between these hormones is mediated between the brain, the uterus, and the ovaries. Many factors, including foreign estrogen in the diet, stress, and intense emotions, can upset this magnificent balance within, as can a prolapsed uterus, which may not send sufficient chemical messages to the brain.

Wild Yam   Mexican wild yam is the herb of choice—it helps the body regulate the menstrual cycle. It is no accident that so many medical doctors prescribe the birth control pill for menstrual irregularity: it is based on a synthetic version of the wild yam.

You need not take the Pill to obtain the benefits of wild yam. This herb is present in many female formulas sold in health food stores and can be taken alone as a tincture. Take one dropper in half a cup of tepid water three times daily.

Osteoporosis

This disease is rare among traditional Maya women. One reason is that the Yucatan Peninsula has some of the most calcium-rich soils in the world. Another reason is that Maya women stay active outdoors all of their lives. Maya women who live in cities and have more means are more susceptible to osteoporosis.

Osteoporosis—which means "porous bones"—occurs mostly in postmenopausal women. Estrogen protects women from bone loss. When estrogen levels decrease, the bones of some women become brittle and easily broken. Normally our bones are rebuilt, remodeled, and replaced regularly, but as we age we lose more bone than we can replace.

Thin women are at a higher risk owing to a paucity of fat cells to act as estrogen storehouses. The Maya believe that menopausal and postmenopausal women should be "pleasantly plump." They believe pleasantly plump women are healthier!

Lack of regular exercise, calcium, and vitamin D from sunshine have been established as primary causes of osteoporosis. Exercise stimulates blood supply to the bones, increasing their mineral content.

The high-calcium foods consumed by the Maya are good for osteoporosis and for everything else related to menopause.

Amaranth Greens and Seeds
Maya women adore amaranth, also known locally as calalu, amaranto, and pigweed. The dark green young leaves are ready to harvest after only three weeks of growth and can be picked for at least two months. The seed heads are gathered when dry, winnowed, roasted, and ground to mix with corn cakes.

ANCIENT WISDOM
The History of Amaranth

Amaranth was sacred to the ancient Maya. Before the Spanish arrived, the Maya made idols to their gods and goddesses carved out of roasted amaranth seeds mixed with human blood. The Spanish outlawed the cultivation of amaranth because they considered the custom barbaric.

Today it is easy to find wild and cultivated amaranth in Maya villages and throughout many parts of the world.

Amaranth greens are eaten boiled, sautéed, added to soups, or added raw to salads. Amaranth is also given as a leaf juice to strengthen women during pregnancy, stop excess menstruation, and increase mother's milk. It's a wonderful tonic for older women.

Purslane Purslane is known to the Maya as *verdalaga* or *xucul* (shoo-cool). Like amaranth, it is a common wild plant found growing just about everywhere. It is revered as a healthy food source that is rich in vitamins, calcium, and a full complement of other minerals that protect, build, and strengthen bones.

Purslane has a delightful, lemony flavor and is added to salads and soups and even pickled with onions. It is a good source of essential fatty acids such as omega-3 and can be substituted for fish oils. It is also a good source of antioxidants.

Avocado Avocados are abundant in Central America. They help us convert calcium into bone mass, just as vitamin D from sunshine does. Some people shun the avocado because of its high fat content, but when eaten with lots of vegetables, as in a green salad or with low-fat cottage cheese, it is a valuable addition to the diet. Don't eat avocados, however, if you have any kind of infection.

> ### FROM THE KITCHEN
> ## Comparing the Calcium Content of Milk and Sesame Seeds
>
> - 100 grams of cow's milk: 119 milligrams of calcium, 87 milligrams of phosphorous
> - 100 grams of sesame seeds: 1,435 milligrams of calcium, 560 milligrams of phosphorous

Sesame Seeds You're talking big-time calcium intake when you regularly include sesame seeds in your diet. They also contain phosphorous, iron, vitamin A, and lots of essential amino acids. Maya women cultivate the seeds because they know how important they are.

Sesame seeds increase mother's milk, reduce symptoms of menopause, gently clean the bowels, and are downright delicious to eat. The Maya make a tasty sesame seed salsa (see page 65).

Painful Intercourse

For information on this condition, see part 3 ("Bodywork").

Premenstrual Syndrome

Maya healers say that women have six senses and men only five. That sixth sense is the ability to be open to the intercession of spiritual forces. A woman's sixth sense is more powerful during menstruation and the premenstrual time. So PMS should stand for "psychic mental superability" rather than "pre-menstrual syndrome." It is not a disease.

The premenstrual woman is experiencing hormonal fluctuations that increase her sensitivity and creativity. In earlier centuries premenstrual and menstruating Maya women, like women in some other cultures, gathered in menstruating huts. There, away from the responsibilities of daily life, they gave each other support during this delicate time. Their extra creativity was valued by the community. During this phase of the month women received dream visions that would inspire, guide, and counsel the entire tribe.

Sadly, this sensitivity and receptivity to the divine has become a lonely burden in modern times. The wisdom of the premenstrual woman no longer garners the respect of men, or even of most other women.

Consider how you can use this time of the month to your advantage. Have a slumber party with girlfriends and see what happens. My bet is that you'll have a great time sharing stories and some very lucid, powerful dreams.

Until the day we once again sit in circle with our sisters, here are some Maya remedies that will help you cope.

Mexican Wild Yam Mexican wild yam is the herb of choice for Maya women who experience discomfort and nervousness before periods. It is easily available at most health food stores.

Wild yam was brought to the attention of modern medicine in the 1930s when the Nahuatl women of southern Mexico were observed eating the young yams as a birth control agent. Wild yam provides diosgenin, from which the birth control pill was eventually synthesized.

Wild Yam Cream Wild yam is now available in cream form. Be sure that you are purchasing a natural remedy and not one containing pharmaceutical progesterone. Rub the cream on the belly a few days before PMS.

Wild Yam Tincture Take one dropper in half a cup of tepid water three times daily for one week before PMS. Wild yam is rich in calcium, which helps stabilize female cycles to control cramping, bloating, and headaches.

Rosemary or Basil Tea Maya women drink rosemary or basil tea for premenstrual blues. It turns out that both basil and rosemary are high in phyto-estrogens, which are known to be beneficial for PMS. Both basil and rosemary are also considered spiritual healing plants by the Maya. It makes sense that they would be used by women at the time of the month when their spiritual awareness is at its peak.

To prepare, place the contents of one packet of fresh supermarket basil or rosemary leaves in two cups of water to boil for five minutes (if using dried leaves, use two teaspoons and boil for ten minutes). Steep for ten minutes. Drink one cup warm before meals two times a day. Use for three days during the premenstrual phase.

Female Tonic Don Elijio used this complex tonic, which includes wild yam root, China root, and ginger (see Resources appendix).

Vaginitis

A young woman of nineteen came to Ix Chel Farm with a distressing case of vaginal itching and discharge. It flared up from time to time but recently had gotten much worse.

Vaginal itching is a side effect of a course of antibiotics that destroys "good" bacteria along with the bad. It is also caused by a prolapsed uterus. As it turned out, this young Maya woman had taken an antibiotic for acne and had a prolapsed uterus.

I adjusted her uterus, suggested she add yogurt to her diet, and gave her some jackass bitters in vinegar to use as a douche. She improved quickly.

Jackass Bitters Douche Soak one tablespoon of dried jackass bitters leaves in half a cup of vinegar overnight. Strain. Add one teaspoon to a cup of water to make the douche.

Pour the mixture into a rubber douching bulb from the drugstore. Douche twice daily. Bottle, label, and store the rest in a cabinet.

The vinegar helps make the environment of the vagina less favorable to the yeast that causes the itching and burning. The jackass bitters destroys the yeast.

If you have vaginitis but haven't taken any antibiotics recently, the uterine massage will do the trick. I once gave a Maya uterine massage to a woman whose vaginitis symptoms cleared up right on the table! Maya midwives tell me that this happens all the time. Once the uterus and cervix are lifted up out of the vaginal canal, the body's own defense forces go right to work.

Physical Ailments of Men

Men came by truck and taxicab, with or without their families, to see Don Elijio. Sometimes they rode in on horseback and tied their horses up under Don Elijio's orange tree.

They usually came to see the old Maya doctor for one of the following reasons—stomach problems, the feeling that "things are not right in my life," or matters of the heart. Others would sheepishly slip in and ask to speak with Don Elijio in private about impotency problems.

In this section you'll learn about the Maya's good, practical remedies for men's physical problems. Turn to part 4 on spiritual illness and healing to learn about remedies for other problems.

Enlarged Prostate

Inflammation of the prostate is known as prostatitis. The swelling or noncancerous enlargement is called benign prostate hyperplasia (BPH). Both occur in men when they hit their forties and fifties. By the age of sixty these conditions are quite common.

The prostate gland is located below the bladder and produces the fluid that transports sperm out of the body. When healthy, the doughnut-shaped gland is about the size of a walnut. An unhealthy prostate can grow to the size of an orange.

Since the urethra, or urinary tube, passes right through the prostate, prostate swelling places abnormal pressure on the urethra.

This causes frequent urination, especially during the night. Other symptoms are burning pain, dribbling urine, and the inability to urinate. Men may also suffer from fevers, backaches, loss of libido, painful ejaculation, and tiredness.

The cause? The jury is still out on the reason for swelling and inflammation of the prostate, but thus far research fingers are pointing at our diets. A modern man's diet is high-fat and low-fiber with too many artificial hormones that stimulate abnormal cellular growth. The average man also consumes too much alcohol and caffeine and doesn't get enough exercise. He sits too much and wears tight underwear and jeans.

This explains why enlarged prostates are not common among Maya men who still follow the traditional ways. They eat indigenous foods such as corn, beans, pumpkins, sesame, fruits, and vegetables. Their diet is high in fiber, and they get plenty of exercise and fresh air.

Prevention   The Maya have some good strategies to prevent the swelling and inflammation of the prostate. Think "seeds" when contemplating prevention of prostate problems.

I have observed that traditional Maya men munch on pumpkin seeds, and even marijuana seeds, "to keep the lines clean and open." "The lines," as I have come to understand, refer to the bladder, prostate, and kidneys.

Munching on seeds has been a habit of Maya men and women for centuries. In addition to pumpkin seeds, they eat sesame seeds, which can be found in many a spicy hot chili salsa.

> ### FROM THE KITCHEN
>
> ### Corn Silk Tea for the Genito-Urinary Tract
>
> Boil the silken hairs of six corn cobs in three cups of water for ten minutes. Drink throughout the day in sips or in half-glass doses.
>
> Maya men don't drink this tea every day, only on occasion, at corn harvest time, or if there is a problem with the "lines."

Seeds contain essential fatty acids and beneficial amounts of zinc, both of which have proven to be important in the prevention of prostate problems.

Pumpkins and their relatives the cucumbers have substances that prevent testosterone from converting to the more harmful dihydrotestosterone (DHT), which stimulates prostate growth.

Another wonderful preventive food is corn, both fresh and ground into tortillas; both are staples of Maya life. Corn is central to Maya physical and spiritual healing. It is a tradition to save the tiny golden hairs of corn cobs to make into a tea that "cleans the lines" of the genito-urinary tract.

Maya men will excitedly exclaim that a lot of "cold" passes when they drink this tea. "Cold" refers to strands of mucus and cloudy urine. They are right to be excited: such passing is an indication that cleansing has occurred.

> ### ANCIENT WISDOM
> #### For Prostate Pain
>
> The Maya use marigold seeds to relieve prostate pain. Boil two dried marigold flower heads (the seeds are in the flower head) and nine leaves in one and a half cups of water for ten minutes. Strain. Drink warm in half-cup doses as needed.

Saw Palmetto The berries of the saw palmetto palm are the most commonly accepted natural remedy for benign prostate enlargement. The Maya also prize it as a remedy for stomach complaints and dysentery.

Scientists believe that the saw palmetto berry weakens the enzyme that triggers prostate growth. Thus far studies have shown no adverse side effects, although it has been noted that the berry tea can cause minor gastrointestinal discomfort.

Saw palmetto berry capsules are available in health food stores everywhere and should be taken according to directions on the label.

Stinging Nettle Root Extract Stinging nettle root is another excellent choice to prevent prostate swelling. This is a common plant that grows throughout the Americas and is used for a variety of common ailments. Don't be fooled by its name—the "stinging" nettle can ease your pain. *Ortiga*, as it is also called, is a plant at the forefront of research.

Studies have shown that extracts of the stinging nettle root can help reduce prostate swelling. A few tablespoons each day can reduce the number of times a man must get up at night to urinate.

The herb may have some inhibitory effect on the conversion of testosterone. According to plant guru Jim Duke in *The Green Pharmacy,* German medical herbalists prescribe two to three tablespoons of extract a day.

Stinging nettles tincture can be purchased at stores that sell herbal remedies, or it can be made at home.

With gloves on, pull up one or two mature plants just before flowering time, preferably after 4:00 P.M. Wash and chop the roots well. Place in a clean glass jar, cover with rum, vodka, or gin, and allow to sit for fourteen days away from sunlight. Label and date jars. Shake once daily. Pour off a few ounces at a time and take two to three tablespoons a day. For store-bought tinctures, take one dropperful three times daily before meals. Nettle root tea takes less time to prepare. For the tea, boil two tablespoons of dried root in three cups of water for ten minutes and steep for twenty minutes and take half a cup three times daily for at least ten days of each month.

Capsules can also be purchased. Take two capsules three times daily before meals or according to instructions on the bottle.

Prostate Massage Probably the most unusual treatment the Maya have to offer is the prostate massage. This external massage of the pelvis stimulates blood flow and helps drain fluids that accumulate and cause swelling. Turn to part 3, "Bodywork," for more information.

Impotency

A Maya farmer who lives down the road from our farm in Belize recently paid me a surprise visit. He arrived on horseback with his two bright-eyed sons riding behind him in the same saddle. I remember thinking that the sight of them—surrounded as they were by palm trees and parrots—would make a beautiful painting.

When the farmer and his boys dismounted, he said that he wanted to talk to me in private. I led him to our thatched-roof clinic and left the little boys on the terrace playing with our dogs.

"It's my nature," the farmer whispered. "Nature," I have learned, always refers to sexual potency. "I can't seem to do it like I used to. I wonder if you have those teas Don Elijio used to give for this. Did you learn that too?"

"First, do you have any other symptoms, like painful urination, backache, fever, or tiredness?" I asked.

"Not really. Nothing more than it won't stay hard, as it used to. I'm only thirty-eight and not ready to give it up yet, and neither is my wife."

"Well then, let's go with Don Elijio's man vine root," I said.

"Right!" he exclaimed excitedly. "That's the one—*behuco de hombre!* You have it?"

"Always keep it on hand," I answered to his growing smile and relief.

I saw him in town the next month and asked how things were going, and he responded with glee, "Todo bien" (All is well).

I don't know of anything that revives male potency as well as the root of man vine from the Maya jungles. Many men report that it does put them on the toilet for a day and give them a good bowel cleansing. Some also say that their urine is cloudy for a day. They know that the cleansing is a good thing and that the results are well worth the minor discomfort.

Man vine is not found beyond the tropics. Check the Resources appendix.

ANCIENT WISDOM
Impotency Prevention Tea

The habit of drinking corn silk tea is common among the Maya. Men say they notice a real difference in sexual performance after a few days of taking three glasses daily. Corn silk works well to prevent impotency because it keeps the genito-urinary tract clean.

ANCIENT WISDOM
Getting Cold Feet

Maya men are quite serious about not walking barefoot on cold surfaces because they say it "cuts the nature." They believe that whatever is cold contracts. A long period of contraction of the muscles of the feet and ankles affects the free flow of blood supply to and from the pelvis. Remember how Anthony Quinn as Zorba the Greek stood on his hands before he made love to his wife?

China Root Something closer to home for treatment of a man's "nature" is the red tuber known as China root or sarsaparilla. This was an original ingredient of root beer.

China root is said to boost testosterone levels in men. It's not wise for men fifty or older to use it: it may stimulate prostate swelling and aggravate existing conditions. China root can be purchased in health food stores and from shops that sell supplies for home brewing.

To prepare, boil three teaspoons of powdered China root in one quart of water for ten minutes. Steep ten minutes. Strain and drink in sips throughout the day. Repeat for three days or until sexual function normalizes.

Back Massage for Impotency A deep muscle tissue massage to the lower back stimulates nerve impulses to the blood vessels of the penis. This is considered standard treatment of impotency by traditional healers. If you wish to try this, you should contact a naprapath, chiropractor, or massage therapist.

Physical Ailments of Infants and Children

The Maya are experts in home remedies for children for good reason. Traditionally a small Maya family is considered one with only *nine* children. A large family can consist of fifteen. This is true even today.

Many of these families live in remote villages, far from modern medical clinics, and so villagers have long relied on each other and the healing knowledge passed down through generations. In general, midwives care for infants while the village healer or family elder cares for children.

So here are some wonderful, natural alternatives to try before you call the doctor about common ailments. Give your kids a break from frequent rounds of synthetic antibiotics and drugs with harmful side effects.

Asthma

Life everlasting is a popular antiwheezing plant that Maya healers prescribe for children and infants because it provides long-term relief. It is said to "ease the breath." (For more information, see "Asthma" in the section on general ailments.)

The sprouted life ever lasting leaves are mashed with a pinch of salt. Extract the juice and give a teaspoon three times daily to children from three months to six years old. Older children can take a tablespoon three times daily.

Known as mother of thousands in the United States and Europe, life everlasting plants can be purchased at most nurseries.

Colic

Not long ago two interns working at our farm fell in love and got married. Soon afterward, baby Gregory was born.

He was a colicky, crabby, sleepless baby, and as every mother knows, such babies are exhausting. Fortunately, my friend Hortence Robinson, the midwife, came to visit a month after his birth. She smiled knowingly as the baby's mother lamented that he woke up every hour on the hour all night long.

Hortence examined the baby. She noticed that his belly was tight and that his little fists doubled up every time he howled, owing, she said, to constipation. She immediately set to work preparing this tea.

Miss Hortence's Tea for Colic with Constipation She boiled a branch of epazote with a three-inch piece of orange rind the size of a finger and a stem of garlic bulb in a cup of water for ten minutes. She used the stem because the garlic bulb is too strong for a baby. (If you make this tea, be sure to open the stem to make sure there are no baby garlics growing inside.)

She strained the tea through a cheesecloth and gave him one ounce every two hours throughout the afternoon—three doses in all. That night he slept four hours at a time. In the light of dawn he awoke with a happy giggle. His diaper was full. From then on he was a happy baby. Occasionally, when he began to complain, his mother repeated the treatment.

Epazote grows wild throughout the Americas. Get to know it. It may be in your yard or just down the street. I recently came across epazote in a Washington, D.C., neighborhood. It's best to use the peel of an organic orange.

Other remedies are used for colic that does not involve constipation.

Allspice Tea Boil together one level teaspoon of allspice berries or half a teaspoon of powdered allspice, one 7-inch-long garlic stem (check for little cloves inside and remove), and one 3-inch piece of organic orange rind (about the width of an adult finger) for ten minutes in a cup of water. Strain well, and give in three 2-ounce doses before nap or bedtime.

Chamomile Flower Tea Infuse one teaspoon of dried chamomile in one cup of water. Strain and give baby one ounce every two hours. Be sure to give three doses before nap or bedtime.

ANCIENT WISDOM

Belly Rub for Baby Colic

This is so helpful and easy to do, and it works great on cranky older children and adults too! Place the baby on her back in a comfortable and well-supported position. Lubricate your fingers with a bit of olive or almond oil and rub lightly on the bare skin between the ribs down to the pelvic area. Stroke downward lightly on both the right and left sides. Then make widening clockwise concentric circles around the belly button. Massage for at least five minutes. This relaxes tight abdominal muscles and relieves gas.

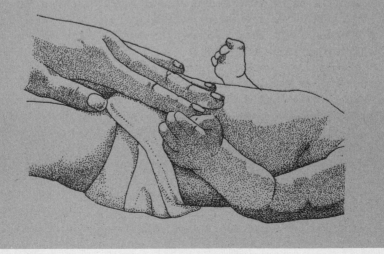

Marigold Flower Tea   This is an all-time favorite of Maya and Aztec women.

Infuse one flower head plus dry skin around a garlic clove (*not* the garlic inside) in one cup of boiling water for twenty minutes. Strain well and give to baby in one-ounce doses every two hours. Be sure baby has three ounces in one day.

Coughs and Colds

Here's my favorite cough syrup for children.

Grannie's Dandelion Cough Syrup

1 qt dandelion flowers, with stems
1 qt water
2 c brown sugar
2 drops eucalyptus oil
2 Tbsp rum

Boil dandelion flowers, stems, water, and brown sugar together for forty-five minutes. Strain and add eucalyptus and rum. Give one teaspoon to smaller children ages one through four every hour. Older children (five to twelve) can take one tablespoon every hour.

The cough syrup will last for many weeks if refrigerated, but it should always be given at room temperature.

FROM THE KITCHEN
Cough Remedy

Here's a Maya remedy for tickling coughs: sip light oatmeal water all day. Boil half a cup of oatmeal in three cups of water for ten minutes, strain, and sweeten with honey. Take in sips throughout the day to soothe the back of the throat. Works for both children and adults.

Phlegm Buster   To loosen the phlegm that comes along with those dry, hacking coughs, boil one tablespoon *each* of dried basil, oregano, and rosemary in three cups of water for ten minutes.

Steep covered for ten minutes. Strain and add the juice of half a lemon and three tablespoons of honey. (Brown sugar is more appropriate for infants as honey can cause infant botulism.) Stir well and give in half-cup doses every two hours during the day. If the child has a fever as well, give the tea as hot as possible. Wrap her up warmly, put her to bed, and let her sweat it out. Be sure to cover the head with a winter cap.

ANCIENT WISDOM
Bullhorn Tree Ants

I know that you can't do this, but it makes for interesting reading. There is an acacia tree in Central America called bullhorn that harbors small, black stinging ants in its thorns. Maya villagers gather nine of these ants and squeeze them in half a cup of water until well mashed up. Then they strain the mixture and give it to infants by the teaspoon for very bad cases of catarrh (mucus). It forces the mucus out of the lungs and sinuses and into the bowels the next day.

Diarrhea

Diarrhea is generally due to something disagreeable in the diet, overeating, or emotional upset. The Maya have a lot of experience treating diarrhea in children and so have a number of household remedies.

FROM THE KITCHEN
Ginger and Lemon for Diarrhea with Stomach Cramps and Vomiting

Grate one tablespoon of fresh ginger and boil in one cup of water for ten minutes. Cover and let sit until room temperature. Add the juice of half a lemon and honey if desired. For small children from ages two to seven, give three tablespoons three times daily. Older children can take three tablespoons every hour until better.

Rice Toast uncooked rice kernels until brown. Boil them without oil in enough water to cover the rice plus one inch. Eat rice (add honey for older children) all day. Blend rice without honey for babies.

Cinnamon Tea Cinnamon tea is always a great aid in alleviating diarrhea. Add a bit of honey, and even the most finicky child will enjoy it. To make, boil a three-inch piece of cinnamon bark or one teaspoon of cinnamon powder in one and a half cups of water.

> **FROM THE KITCHEN**
> **Red Rose Tea for Baby Diarrhea**
> Boil one red rose with six inches of leaves and stem in one cup of water for five minutes. Steep tea until cooled to room temperature. Strain. Give one ounce to infants up to twelve months old three times during the day. For babies from thirteen months to three years, give two ounces three times a day. Repeat for two to three days if necessary.

Boil for ten minutes. Steep until cool. Strain and add a teaspoon of honey. Drink in two half-cup doses over one hour.

Bananas and Applesauce The Maya give children with loose bowels only ripe bananas all day. Applesauce works well too. The same goes for adults.

Drinking Lots of Fluids Be sure to give lots of fluids in the form of water and fruit juices to replace water and electrolyte loss.

Ear Infections

In the United States, ear infections are the primary reason parents bring children to see a doctor. Caused by a combination of lack of breast-feeding, proximity to other children with infections, and genes, they are all too common. So, unfortunately, is the treatment of choice—antibiotics. Even antibiotics don't end the cycle. Many ear infections flare up again as soon as the drugs wear off.

I'm pleased to tell you that ear infections pose no difficulty for Maya healers. I've learned two terrific and easy treatments to pass on to you. These Maya home remedies work as well for adults as for children.

First gather or buy fresh leaves of either oregano, thyme, or basil. Warm a quarter-cup of the leaves over a low flame in a dry skillet until the leaves are limp, not burned. Don't overcook.

When the leaves are cool enough to hold, squeeze them between your fingers over the ear opening. Holding the head to the side, let three to five drops of the leaf juice fall into the ear.

Then lubricate your fingers with a bit of olive oil and rub the side of the neck around the painful ear. Between two protruding bones behind the ear, you will find little, hard, painful bumps—the

clogged lymph nodes, which are preventing drainage from the ear and allowing bacteria and pus to accumulate. To help them drain, press the bumps with downward strokes as hard as can be tolerated for one to five minutes. The longer the better. Do the same thing behind the other ear. Repeat this treatment at three-hour intervals throughout the day. It really works.

Olive Oil and Garlic Variation In a blender combine a quarter-cup of olive oil with one chopped medium-sized clove of garlic for one minute. Pour off and heat until the mixture is warm. Dip the tip of a sterile cotton ball into the mixture and place inside the painful ear. Massage both sides of the neck as above. Keep the cotton in the ear during the massage. Replace with a fresh application of olive oil and garlic three times daily. Bottle and label the mixture to store for future use.

Fever

Fevers are a completely natural and common part of childhood. A child's immune system needs a chance to fight off bacteria and other harmful invaders. If a fever is below 102 degrees Fahrenheit, it is usually okay to use home remedies. If the fever is higher than 102 degrees or there is any sign of convulsions, seek medical assistance immediately.

By the way, feverish children are usually not hungry. They want only fluids. Forced feeding can lead to indigestion and compound their illness. A light vegetable soup or fruit juice, especially orange juice, is more than enough.

The Maya have several wonderful fever remedies for children.

Lemongrass Tea Lemongrass (also known as fever grass) is the herb of choice among Maya villagers. How lucky that it tastes like candy when sweetened! Lemongrass can be purchased dried in Spanish and Asian grocery stores.

> ### ANCIENT WISDOM
> #### Aloe on the Feet
>
> I've seen Maya midwives break off pieces of an aloe plant and wrap them around the child's feet to draw down the fever. Clean the aloe of any thorns that might scratch the baby, then slice the aloe in half lengthwise. Lightly bind to the feet with cotton cloth or use socks to hold in place. As the fever is drawn out of the body the aloe dries up. Replace it with fresh pieces.

Boil a small handful of the dried stems (as much as fits in the palm of your hand) in a cup of water for ten minutes. Strain, add sugar, and give to the child as warm as possible. Wrap the child up warmly and allow him to sweat freely.

Marigold or Basil Bath This works wonders. Boil a quart of marigold flowers or basil leaves in a big pot of water. Cover pot and steep until the water is warm, not hot. Pour into bathwater and let the child play. Don't let her get chilled after the bath.

Purges Maya mothers believe that it's good to give a laxative when a baby's fever is high and persistent. Miss Hortence's baby colic tea made of epazote, orange rind, and garlic stem (see under "Colic") works well as a fever purge. Purges also work for feverish older children. The Maya use an indigenous plant they call *xcoch*—otherwise known as castor bean! A generous teaspoon of that infamous castor oil works wonders for older children.

Skin Infections

Years ago, shortly after I began working with Don Elijio, a four-year-old and her parents showed up in his clinic. They had traveled all the way from Guatemala City, a journey of several days. She was sickly and pale with chronic, infected sores all over her body.

This was one of the most dramatic cures I ever saw Don Elijio accomplish. First, he bathed her three times a day in hot water in which he had boiled jackass bitters. Then, while the sores were still wet, he applied a powder of dried jackass bitters. He also gave the child a purge to clean out her bowels.

FROM THE KITCHEN
Boils

I wish my mother had known about these boil remedies used by my Maya neighbors. I used to get painful boils on my backside that made it impossible to go to school because I couldn't sit. Here are a few old-time recipes to draw boils.

Black Beans Soak half a cup of raw black beans in two cups of water overnight. Blend the following morning with just enough water to make a paste, and add half a teaspoon of olive or almond oil. Apply this on a piece of gauze to the boil until it feels as if it is pulling. Replace three times daily until the boil comes out.

Soap and Brown Sugar Grate a tablespoon of Lux (or Ivory) hand soap and add a teaspoon of brown sugar. Mix it well and apply the mixture to a piece of gauze to use as a poultice over the boil. Change the dressing three times daily until the boil comes out.

Within two weeks her sores vanished and her health and spirit had been restored. She didn't seem like the same child.

Herbal Bath You need very bitter plants for this treatment. I recommend the leaves of motherwort, wormwood, or dandelion. Use one or any combination of two or all three.

Boil a quart of the leaves in two quarts of water for twenty minutes. Wash the infection with the water as hot as possible—take care not to burn the skin. Test the temperature with your elbow first. If it's too hot for your elbow to bear, it's too hot to use on a child. Use only warm water for diabetic children.

> ### ANCIENT WISDOM
> ### Mother's Milk and Bread
>
> Mash one tablespoon of mother's milk with a small piece of bread until you make a nice, soft, wet mush. Apply as with the bean and sugar-soap remedies to draw boils.

Wound Powder for Infected Sores Jackass bitters is the ingredient of first choice, but if it is not available to you (see Resources appendix on how to order) or if you need something quickly, here's what to do. You can use basil leaves, dandelion leaves, Saint-John's-wort, vervain, or motherwort.

Take half a cup of dried leaves of any two or three of these plants. Remove stems and leaf veins. Place in a dry skillet over a low to medium flame and stir continuously with a wooden spoon until the leaves are very dry and starting to smoke. When the leaves are cool enough, rub them through a strainer and collect the fine powder in a clean dish. Store in a clean, dry jar, label, and date. Sprinkle over wounds after having washed with any of the herbal bath formulas for skin infections. Alternatively, you can wash with soap and water, apply castor oil to the wound, and then sprinkle on the wound powder. Cover with a clean cotton cloth. Change the dressing twice daily.

Skin Rashes

Skin rashes are very common in infants, and they are often caused by an adverse reaction to food. Maya mothers usually avoid this by feeding babies breast milk and fruits until they are a year old. Other causes may be laundry soap or emotional tension in the household.

Extra water intake and herbal baths are the classic Maya treatments.

Herbal Baths You need a quart of one of the following, or a combination of any three: fresh marigold flowers; basil leaves; hibiscus flowers and/or leaves; red roses; vervain leaves and/or flowers.

Boil the flowers and leaves in a large pot in two gallons of water for ten minutes. Let sit until the water is warm, not hot. Strain and pour into baby's bathwater.

Let the baby soak and play for half an hour. Pour some of the bathwater onto her back and head every few minutes. If the baby is unable to sit up, hold her in the water for at least twenty minutes, pouring cups of the bathwater over her head. Take care not to get bathwater directly into her eyes.

> ## QUICK RELIEF
> ### Corn Starch
> If the rash is due to summer heat, corn starch can be applied lightly two or three times daily. Cooling baths with herbs will also help. The water should be just below room temperature.

Let the skin air-dry or lightly pat her dry. Take care not to let her get chilled after the bath. Wrap her warmly in a towel. She will sleep deeply after this bath.

Newborn Flower Bath For newborn babies with rashes, red roses or red hibiscus are the best flowers to use. Prepare as above with nine red roses or nine red or pink hibiscus flowers. If no flowers are on the bush, use a handful of leaves and six inches of stem. Boil in a gallon of water for ten minutes. Be sure the water is room temperature before you bathe the baby.

Sleeplessness

Not all sleeping problems of babies are caused by colic. Some just won't sleep well, period. Absolutely the best cure for sleepless babies is an herbal bath plus two ounces of either chamomile or catnip tea. When my daughter, Crystal, was an infant and wouldn't sleep more than fifteen minutes at a time, I bathed her in marigold flowers and leaves and gave her the two ounces of chamomile tea. She slept so soundly that I went to check whether she was still breathing.

Chamomile or Catnip Tea Add a teaspoon of either chamomile flowers or catnip leaves to a cup of hot water. Steep for ten minutes. Strain and give two ounces before nap or bedtime.

Sleeplessness in older children is less common. Most kids usually fall asleep anywhere, anytime. But if sleeplessness becomes a problem, I recommend an herbal bath for two or three nights before bedtime. Children love herbal baths and have a grand time helping with the collection and preparation. After the bath they are lighter emotionally and much calmer.

I remember the six-year-old son of a close friend who was emotionally burdened by his parents' divorce. One stressful day we bathed him in white roses, hollyhocks, basil, marigold, and rosemary. I wish you could have seen the light-hearted, happy, playful little boy skipping down the street afterward. It was delightful to see him so light again. That night he slept like a baby.

For more information, read about the sensitive plant under "Insomnia" in the section on general physical ailments.

Garlic, known as "poor man's penicillin," was used successfully during World War I to

Natural Antibiotics

Antibiotics seem to be modern medicine's prescription for everything from ear infections to vaginitis. For generations, however, traditional healers have successfully used a number of alternatives to synthetic antibiotics, and with good reason. Our bodies need time to respond to an infection, and we shouldn't interfere too soon. Additionally, invading organisms often develop immunities of their own to synthetic antibodies, becoming resistant to standard medical treatment.

Natural Antibiotics for Internal Infections

Garlic No doubt the most famous universal infection fighter is garlic. Maya traditional healers in Belize highly respect garlic's ability to fight infection in patients of all ages.

treat infected wounds and amoebic dysentery. Along with onions and chives, garlic is rich in antiseptic and immune system-boosting compounds. It contains allicin, sulfur-containing essential oils, and vitamins A, B, C, D, and E. It is antibacterial, antifungal, anti-inflammatory, antimicrobial, and antiparasitic. It is hypotensive, which means it reduces blood pressure. And as an expectorant, it loosens phlegm.

Garlic can be used in various ways to fight infection. The easiest thing to do is to purchase garlic oil capsules from the store or pharmacy. The standard dose for treating an infection is two garlic capsules three times daily for adults and half that for children ages six to twelve.

FROM THE KITCHEN
Garlic Remedies

Fresh garlic preparations can be made ahead of time and kept on hand in the kitchen.

Honey-Garlic Chop one entire head of raw garlic with skins. Soak in one pint of honey overnight. Take one teaspoon of the honey three times daily for adults and two times daily for children.

Olive Oil–Garlic Prepare as above but in a pint of olive oil. Dosage is the same as for honey-garlic.

Raw Garlic If you're a stalwart, you can just chop up garlic on your food. Consume six to ten cloves a day depending on your size.

Jackass Bitters The highly respected jackass bitters, also known as *tres puntas,* is antibacterial, antifungal, antiparasitic, and antimicrobial. It is intensely bitter, so it is usually prepared in a tincture with alcohol so that you can consume a lot less of it to achieve the same effect. One tablespoon of a tincture provides the same benefit as one cup of tea (see Resources appendix).

Gumbo-limbo Bark Another wonderful tropical alternative to synthetic antibiotics is the red gumbo-limbo bark. Research by the ethnobotanist Janice Alcorn has shown that this much-loved tree bark has an antibiotic substance in its clear resin. Gumbo-limbo is pleasant-tasting, especially when brewed with cinnamon. It makes a tea that even the most finicky child will enjoy. Drink three cups daily.

Gumbo-limbo trees grow in some southern and western states (see Resources appendix).

Natural Antibiotics for Skin Infections

Chamomile Flowers Chamomile flowers are an effective antibacterial agent and wound healer.

Boil a large handful (what will fit into one pint jar) of dried chamomile flowers in two gallons of water for five minutes. Strain, then use to wash infected wounds and sores. Pour the room-temperature herbal water over the affected area three times daily. Let the herbal water air-dry on the skin. If the infection is large or hard to reach, soak the affected part in a tub or basin for thirty minutes.

If fresh plants are available, boil two or three entire plants for five minutes in two gallons of water. Let sit for twenty minutes before using.

This treatment is safe for babies, children, adults, and the elderly. There are no known negative side effects from chamomile blossoms.

Basil If you are lucky enough to have basil growing in your garden, you possess a veritable medicine chest. Isola, my Italian grandmother, used to grow it

FROM THE KITCHEN
Basil Remedies

Basil Rinse For skin infections, boil three large branches about twelve to eighteen inches in length in two gallons of water for ten minutes. Steep for twenty minutes and let cool to room temperature. Use as a rinse three times daily.

Basil Powder If the infection doesn't show signs of healing in three days, here's what to do. Oven-dry the fresh basil leaves at 150 degrees Fahrenheit for about forty-five minutes. Crush well and pass through a tea strainer to make a fine powder. Remove stems and any large pieces.

After bathing in the basil water, pour a bit of castor oil over the wounds, then sprinkle the basil powder over the sores. Apply a sterile wrapping. Repeat twice daily.

on the back porch of her apartment building in Chicago. Not only did she grow it for pesto and tomato sauce, but she prized it as a useful household herb. Maya women also honor this common herb and sometimes call it "holy basil."

The various essential oils in basil that are responsible for its distinctive, inviting aroma are antibacterial and antifungal.

Beef Lard and Honey During the l970s I lived in a remote Nahuatl Indian village in the Sierra Madre in southern Mexico. One of the village elders was a beekeeper who prepared a healing ointment for sores and skin infections.

One day I went to visit her and asked her to show me how to make this salve. "Es facil!" she exclaimed (It's easy!). She mixed three teaspoons of beef lard with one teaspoon of honey until it was a smooth consistency. As she mixed, she explained that her grandmother had taught her this recipe, which "draws water from germs to kill them on the site." The salve also prevented bandages and dressings from sticking to wounds.

She made me a gift of the ointment, which she wrapped into a corn skin tied with a strip of vine that she pulled off of a plant growing on her verandah. Later that week I had the opportunity to try it on my six-year-old son's scraped and infected knee. After three applications over thirty-six hours, his knee healed nicely.

Other "Antibiotic" Plants Skin infections can also be treated with marigold, oregano, dandelion, thyme, or sage.

PART III

Maya Bodywork
and Massage

Maya massage techniques are almost unknown but may be the most ingenious gift they have to offer modern health care.

Traditional healers throughout the world have always used massage therapy techniques, usually learned from parents and grandparents. What distinguishes the Maya is that they still practice the now-forgotten abdominal massage, which, according to Native American lore, is "as old as the world."

Most massage therapists are afraid to touch the abdomen and pelvis. They are often taught during training to avoid these areas entirely. In contrast, Maya healers usually focus their entire treatment on the abdomen.

Perhaps the abdomen is taboo in modern massage therapy training because it is the storehouse of so many human emotions. Unexpressed emotions like fear, anger, and resentment tighten muscle fibers around the arteries and organs, blocking blood flow. Since life energy, the ch'ulel, is in the blood, energy flow is also blocked. Interestingly, the stomach corresponds to the solar plexus chakra, and the pelvis to the kundalini chakra. Maya massage reopens blocked energy paths and releases negative ch'ulel that has accumulated owing to unexpressed emotions.

I had never heard of Maya massage until I met Don Elijio. As a naprapath, I did know a lot about bodywork. Naprapathy, an offshoot of chiropractic medicine, is a system of gentle manipulation intended to normalize the flow of blood, lymph, and nerve function and to repair connective tissue damage.

So I was fascinated to see what Don Elijio could do with his hands. He had a cute little wooden chair that he had made especially for abdominal massage. Patients sat comfortably in a position that made it easy for Don Elijio to reach their abdomen. There was nothing embarrassing or private about an abdominal massage. He massaged men, women, and children alike in a hut without walls, talking and joking the whole time.

He used massage on gastrointestinal complaints of every imaginable type, prostate problems, varicose veins, backaches, and a wide variety of women's complaints. The most sought after technique was the centering of the uterus. He was famous for his ability to alleviate female troubles by centering the prolapsed or tipped uterus.

Eventually Don Elijio taught me how to perform these preventive and therapeutic techniques. I have come to value them as perhaps the greatest and most unappreciated gift of the Maya.

In this part of the book you will learn basic Maya self-help bodywork techniques for men, women, and children. I have been training laypeople and health practitioners alike in the use of these techniques for over a decade.

Self-help workshops are offered throughout the year in which men and women are taught to perform the abdominal massage on themselves and their partners. There is also an advanced certification program for practitioners (see Resources appendix).

As always, if you are having a problem, go see a doctor, but it makes sense to try these simple noninvasive external massage techniques before drugs, surgery, or other invasive procedures.

Maya Massage for Women

Don Elijio believed that a woman's center is her uterus. "If a woman's uterus is out of balance, so is she," he would say. Ch'ulel emanates from the uterus, the seat of creation.

Midwives and healers agree that most female troubles are caused by a wandering womb. Normally the uterus leans slightly over the bladder in the center of the pelvis—about one and a half inches above the pubic bone. It is held in this position by muscles, the vaginal wall, and ligaments that attach it to the back, front, and sides of the pelvis.

Uterine ligaments are made to stretch to accommodate a growing fetus inside and to move freely when the bladder or bowel is full. The ligaments and muscles can weaken and loosen, causing the uterus to fall downward, forward, backward, or to either side. A uterus in any of these positions is called prolapsed or tipped.

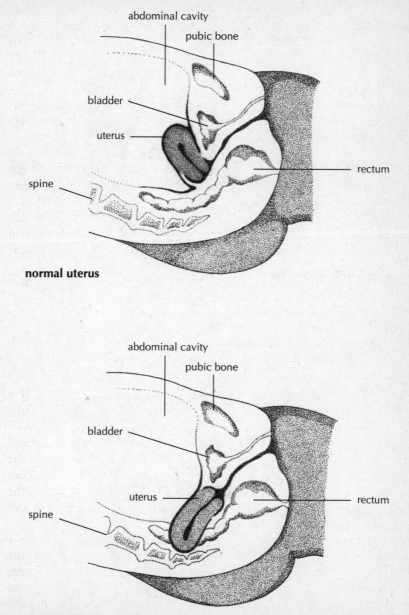

abdominal cavity

pubic bone

bladder

uterus

spine

rectum

normal uterus

abdominal cavity

pubic bone

bladder

uterus

spine

rectum

uterus with retroversion

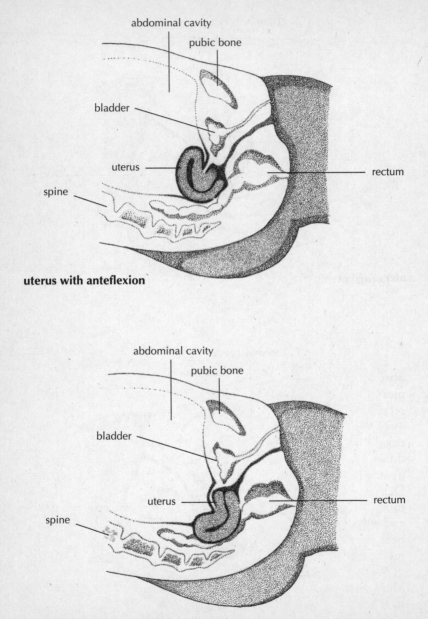

uterus with anteflexion

uterus with anteflexion with retroversion

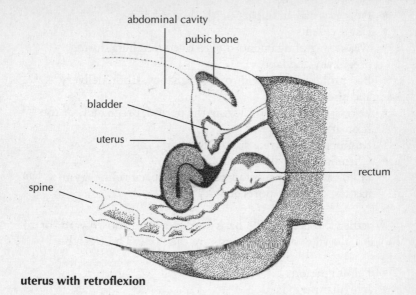

uterus with retroflexion

Seventy-five percent of women have a wandering womb that obstructs the free flow of fluids through this part of the body. This means that that the uterus, ovaries, bladder, and bowel are not receiving sufficient blood or life energy.

Untold numbers of hysterectomies could be prevented with this simple, easy-to-learn, and safe massage technique. When done properly, external, noninvasive massage strengthens the ligaments and muscles that support the uterus and ovaries. Depending on the severity of the problem, it may take a few minutes or a few months for the uterus to slide back into place and stay there. In some women the damage to the ligaments has been so severe that correction is no longer possible by this method.

Women who have had hysterectomies benefit greatly from Maya uterine massage as well. The technique improves circulation in and around the area of the scar.

Some causes of a prolapsed uterus are these:

- Falls that had an impact on the lower back
- Car accidents
- Weakening of ligaments due to overstretching during pregnancy and labor
- Bad professional care during pregnancy, labor, delivery, and afterward
- Carrying heavy loads during the period, pregnancy, or too soon after delivery
- Running on concrete surfaces
- Chronic constipation
- High-impact dancing, aerobics, horseback riding, gymnastics, or other sports activity

Whether the uterus falls backward, forward, downward, or to the sides, the signs and symptoms are the same. There can be

- Painful periods
- Irregular periods
- Dark, thick fluids at the beginning and end of the period
- Blood clots
- No menstruation at all
- Headaches
- Dizziness
- Varicose veins
- Tired legs, numb feet, and sore heels
- Lower backache
- Infertility
- Endometritis
- Endometriosis
- Polyps
- Painful intercourse
- PMS
- Uterine infections
- Frequent urination
- Ovarian cysts
- Vaginitis
- Hormonal imbalances
- Difficult pregnancy and delivery

- Difficult menopause
- Cancer of the cervix, uterus, colon, or bladder

A slim and active forty-two-year-old woman came to see me while I was in the United States on a lecture tour. She had one child, age twelve, and would have loved to have another, but that was not the main reason for her visit.

Ever since she had started to menstruate at age eleven she had experienced severe cramping on the first two days. The cramps were powerful enough to keep her in bed for two days every month. Since she was a schoolteacher, this made her life very difficult.

She also complained of painful intercourse, recurrent vaginitis, and PMS. No one had ever been able to diagnose the problem.

Our discussion revealed that she had slammed her backside on a log when she was six. The area between her legs was black and blue for weeks afterward.

When I examined her, I could see that her uterus was extremely low, and probably had been since that fall. I performed the Maya uterine massage on her and then taught her how to do daily follow-up massages. I also prescribed an herbal formula for ten days before each period for three months.

She wrote four months later to report that all of her symptoms had disappeared. The improvement had been gradual but sure, and she was now confident and comfortable with the massage techniques. She was even teaching her sister and daughter.

Everything was fine, she said, until she moved to a new house and neglected her massage routine at the same time. After three days of carrying heavy items, her old symptoms began to return. Once she started the daily massages again, her symptoms improved quickly.

Do not perform the Maya uterine massage on yourself if

- You have had abdominal surgery within the last six months
- You are under medical treatment for cancer or pelvic abdominal infection
- You are pregnant

- You experience intense pain or discomfort during the self-care massage that does not decrease with each successive treatment
- You are taking painkillers or any medication that may mask discomfort during treatment
- You begin to have intense emotional upheavals during or after the massage treatment (you need to be with someone who can help you with emotional healing)
- Your period is due within five days
- You are experiencing sudden onset of abdominal pain and have not yet been evaluated by a physician
- You have an IUD (intra-uterine device for birth control)

Instructions for Self-Care Uterine Massage

Anyone can learn Maya uterine massage. Wear loose clothing with no zippers. Trim your fingernails. It is probably best to have a friend read the instructions to you as you perform these techniques. By the way, the best time to massage your uterus is anytime after menstruation up until five days before your next period.

Finding Your Uterus It's not as difficult as you might think.
Start by emptying your bladder.
Lie down on your back in a comfortable position with a pillow under your knees. Relax and breathe deeply for a few minutes.

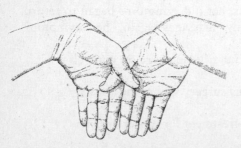

The uterus lies in the middle of your pelvis below the belly button, just above the pubic bone. The pubic bone is the prominent bone between your upper thighs. If in its proper position, the uterus lies about one and a half inches above that bone and is centered in the middle of the pelvis.

Place your two hands together with the thumbs tucked behind the index fingers out of the way.

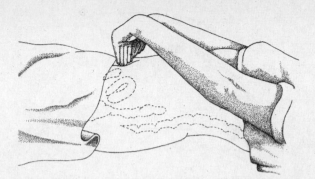

Locate the pubic bone and place the fingertips of both hands on it.

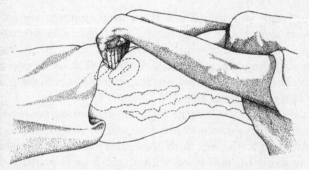

Feel around with your fingers for a slight indentation in the middle of the bone.

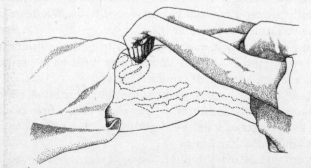

When you find it, place both of your index fingers on that indentation and align your other fingers along the pubic bone in a comfortable position.

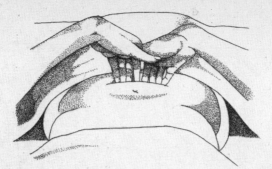

Now slowly slide your hands into the soft flesh above the bone moving toward the belly button.

If your hands sink in and you feel a deep empty space with the pubic bone now above your hands, your uterus is probably in proper position. If so, it is still advisable to perform the massage techniques on yourself to stimulate the flow of blood in and out of the pelvis. This is good prevention. Stagnant fluids collecting in this area can lead to problems later.

If your uterus doesn't seem to be in the proper position, you will quickly feel resistance to pressure and be unable to sink your fingers deeply into the soft flesh above the pubic bone. It will feel something like a balloon filled with water. This is probably your prolapsed uterus.

Performing the Massage Don't get frustrated or overwhelmed. It doesn't really matter if you can't locate your uterus. Wherever it is, the massage treatment is the same.

Still lying on your back, move the pillow from under your knees to under your buttocks. Bend your knees. Breathe deeply and slowly for a few minutes until you feel relaxed.

Bring both of your hands together onto the pubic bone, tucking one thumb under the other with the eight other fingers close together. Your fingers should be slightly bent and relaxed so that your two hands look like a hoe.

Slide your hands off the pubic bone toward your head and sink your fingers as deep as you comfortably can into the soft flesh.

Dig deeply here, as long as you do not feel any pain. If you experience pain, lighten up, but don't give up. Keep massaging as deeply as is comfortable for you in an upward motion toward the belly button.

Ignore the resistance you feel—just slide right over it and keep massaging upward. Go back to the pubic bone and start again. Repeat this movement from pubic bone to belly button for two minutes.

If you experience pain or discomfort, lighten up on the pressure but continue to massage upward and as deeply as you can within the comfort zone. If pain persists even with a lighter touch, stop. At this point you should be examined and evaluated by a qualified health-care practitioner or a professional trained in these massage techniques (to find such a therapist, see Resources appendix).

Women who have had hysterectomies or C-sections may feel some lumpy, hard scar tissue just above the pubic bone. Sometimes this is painful owing to poor circulation in the area around the scar. As long as the discomfort is not severe, continue with the self-care massage. The pain should diminish little by little. If it doesn't, stop and consult with a health-care practitioner.

After the Massage   If you are tender to the touch the following day, you have been massaging too deeply. Lighten up and give your uterus a few days' rest.

Otherwise, repeat the massage the next day and every day thereafter for one minute at a time once a day. Breathe slowly while counting to sixty. The best time to do a self-care abdominal massage is when you get into bed at night or just before arising in the morning. You know which one works best for you.

Don't be distressed that you may not be performing this technique correctly. Just follow the instructions to the best of your ability. Each day you will become more familiar with the massage and more confident of your touch.

What You May Experience After This Treatment   Most women report that they feel a distinctive improvement in the circulation throughout their pelvis, legs, and feet during and after the treatment. They often describe it as feeling "much lighter." Observers witness a healthy flush of colors in the cheeks, often described as "glowing." Some women say that they can see and think more clearly.

Once your uterus is in place and the ligaments have begun to heal enough to hold it there permanently, you may experience some changes in your menstruation, including more blood flow, darker fluids, and a temporary increase in the number of days you flow. Some women experience a spontaneous off-cycle period. Don't worry—this is a sign that your uterus is getting healthy again. Gradually, over about three months, your period will return to or become normal. If it doesn't, or if you feel worried, contact a trained therapist for advice (see the Resources appendix).

When to Perform Self-Care Massage   Perform the self-care massage every day for thirty days, then twice a week thereafter. Stop five days before your period is due. If you are irregular and don't know when it is due, continue the massage until it flows. When your period is over, continue again. Although not generally recommended, some women find that a *light* uterine massage gives relief from menstrual cramps.

If you have a lot of female troubles or are infertile and would like to conceive, perform the self-care massage daily every cycle for three months, then three times weekly after that.

Perform this massage after you have lifted heavy things, fallen, gone running, or taken a high-impact aerobics class. Dancers and athletes should perform the self-care massage daily for their entire career. In just one minute a day they can prevent a lifetime of reproductive problems.

Maya Massage for Men

Men benefit from Maya abdominal massage techniques too. By ensuring a full blood supply to the prostate, the abdominal massage helps to prevent swelling and inflammation. My male patients report that they can feel a distinct difference in blood flow before and after a treatment. Not only does the Maya massage relieve prostate swelling, but it helps alleviate varicose veins, premature ejaculation, some impotency problems, and the need to urinate frequently.

A fifty-year-old American expatriate came to my clinic to ask whether I had anything to help with circulation.

"Why do you ask?" I queried.

"Well, lately I've noticed that the veins in my lower legs and feet are very big and ropy. They weren't like that before, and I just thought it would be good to get something so it doesn't get worse."

"Have you been urinating frequently lately?" I asked.

"Oh, yes, but mostly at night, which, come to think of it, is new to me also. What's going on?"

"Well, since you are fifty now, we need to consider that it might be swelling in the prostate slowing the flow of blood in the veins."

I examined him and detected some soreness around the prostate. I performed the Maya massage for ten minutes, then taught him how to do the self-care massage. He was to do it twice a day for one minute. The easiest time would be before getting in and out of bed.

When he got up from the treatment table, the varicose veins in his feet were clearly less prominent. I also gave him some Maya herbs and told him to be sure to drink at least eight glasses of water daily (see "Enlarged Prostate" in the men's physical ailments section of part 2).

A few weeks later I saw him at a party, and he was proud to show me that the veins in his feet were back to normal. At most, he was getting up now once a night to urinate. He made me laugh when I asked him whether he found it tiresome or difficult to do the massage. "Oh, no!" he said, "I taught my girlfriend to do it for me."

Instructions for Prostate Massage

Don't perform this massage if

- You have had abdominal surgery within the last six months
- You are under medical treatment for cancer or pelvic abdominal infection
- You experience intense pain or discomfort during the self-care massage that does not diminish with each treatment
- You are taking painkillers or any medication that may mask discomfort during the treatment

- You begin to have intense emotional upheavals during or after the massage treatment (you need to be with someone who can help you to pass through the gates of emotional healing)
- You are experiencing sudden onset of abdominal pain and have not yet been evaluated by a physician

Performing the Massage Wear comfortable loose clothing. This means no blue jeans and no zippers. Empty your bladder.

Lie in a comfortable place with a pillow under the buttocks and bend the knees.

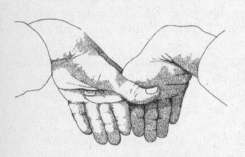

Breathe deeply for a few minutes until you feel relaxed.

Bring both of your hands together, tucking one thumb under the other and bring all eight fingers close together, slightly bent and relaxed so that your hands form what looks like a garden hoe.

There is a prominent bone between your thighs called the pubic bone. See if you can locate it with your two hands held together as described. When you do, feel around with your index fingers for a slight indentation in the middle of the bone.

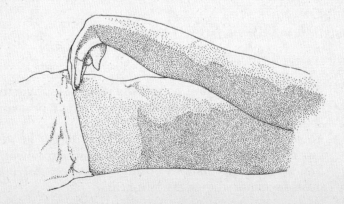

Place both of your index fingers on the indentation and align your other fingers along the pubic bone.

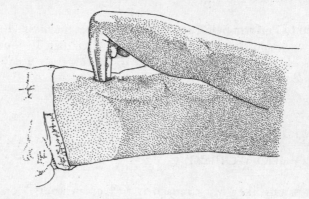

Now slide all eight fingers off the bone, keeping your thumbs well tucked out of the way.

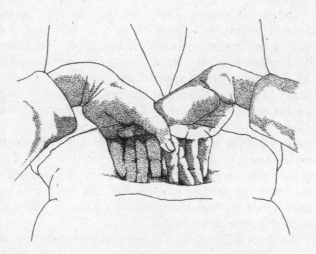

You may be able to sink your fingers quite deeply into the soft tissue above this bone with no discomfort or resistance. As long as you do not feel pain, pull the flesh upward toward the belly button and jiggle slightly from side to side maintaining your deep pressure the entire time.

Repeat this upward movement from pubic bone to belly button for one minute. You can count to sixty slowly while breathing deeply to mark the time.

When to Perform Self-Care Massage Repeat the massage daily for one week and then three times weekly after that. If you are fifty years old or over, it's a good idea to do this once a day for one minute.

Abdominal Massage for Both Men and Women

Expressions like "My stomach is tied up in knots," or, "I can't stomach her," have their origin in physical reality. The Maya address this reality by performing massage that is focused on the upper abdomen.

The abdominal massage involves the abdomen above and around the belly button. Because the anatomy of men and women is the same in this region, these instructions apply to both sexes.

Abdominal massage can help alleviate gastritis, indigestion, constipation, heartburn, lack of appetite, and the feeling of tightness in the stomach. I do the self-care stomach massage every single day and find that it helps my occasional bouts of nervous stomach and indigestion.

It is also good for my emotional equilibrium. Abdominal massage can release the deep-seated emotions that underlie many chronic stomach complaints that are considered incurable. Often patients with long-standing gastritis are nervous, high-strung, or depressed. Once the chronic stomach spasm is relaxed, these patients feel better within minutes.

Practitioners of Chinese medicine often perform upper abdominal massage. Releasing the muscular tension of the diaphragm muscle allows the digestive organs to function properly, alleviates constipation, and helps prevent a host of digestive and intestinal problems. It also releases the energy of blocked life force.

The same precautions apply to the upper abdominal massage as to the lower (see page 143).

Performing Upper Abdominal Massage

Lie on your back in a comfortable position, with a pillow under the knees. Breathe deeply and slowly a few minutes until you relax.

Hold your hands together in the position shown in the illustration on page 144.

Place the hands on the flesh between the rib cage. Apply direct pressure by moving your hands back and forth in a downward motion toward the belly button. When you reach the belly button, you may feel some pain. Lighten up but don't give up. With the fingertips of both hands, make deep pressing movements around the belly button clockwise.

Do this for two minutes.

Varicose Veins

The Maya abdominal massage can make a real difference. Most varicose veins in women are due to a prolapsed uterus preventing the free flow of blood toward the heart from the legs. A swollen prostate can also cause varicose veins.

Massage for Children

Touch is a wonderful healing tool for children, most of whom love it. One midwife I know performs massage on newborn infants daily for nine days. "That way they don't give trouble," she says confidently. All children benefit from massage. It is especially helpful for anxiety, headaches, nail biting, growing pains, stomach troubles, overstimulation, and sleep disorders.

Getting Started

Choose a massage oil. I recommend almond, calendula, grapeseed, or jojoba. There are some lovely, smooth blends available from stores. It's nice to include a soothing aromatic essential oil such as lavender, rose, orange, or chamomile. (Choose one that you use all the time—your child will learn to associate pleasant memories with that fragrance.) Place one drop of essential oil in each ounce of massage oil. Don't overdo it. Shake well.

Infant Massage

If possible, bathe the infant in either plain warm water or an herbal bath. Heat the oil so it is slightly warm.

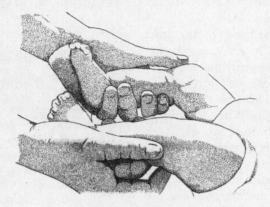

Lay the baby on her back. Gently massage a few drops of oil on her feet and calves, taking care not to apply too much pressure. Spend five minutes massaging the legs and feet.

In long even strokes, work your way up the trunk toward the head. Massage the arms and hands in an upward motion toward the heart for five minutes. Take care that the baby doesn't get oil on her hands, which she could rub into her eyes. Wipe her hands with a dry washcloth every few minutes to be extra careful.

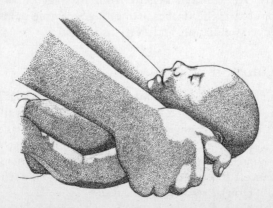

Turn the baby over on her tummy. Starting at the buttocks, massage the back up to the neck in the same long even strokes for five minutes.

Turn the baby over again. Focus now on her head and neck. Hold her head in your hands and using your fingertips, *gently* rub the base of her skull for two minutes. Massage her face in light circular motions around the forehead, cheeks, and chin.

Now to the belly. With a very light touch, make several clockwise circles around the belly button.

Finish off with another light foot massage to ensure good circulation.

Wrap her up warmly. Feed her if the timing is right, and enjoy her coos and smiles before she takes a long, peaceful nap.

Children's Massage

Because some children may not be willing to participate out of fear of the unknown, I always demonstrate what I am about to do on a doll—without the oil, of course. Kids love it. I place the doll on the massage table and perform a light and quick massage, then invite them up to the table. It almost always works. A regular or herbal bath beforehand will help them relax.

Once the child is ready, follow the general instructions for infant massage. You can apply a bit more pressure for older children, but not much more.

"Tell me if it hurts," I tell them. That way they know that you are tuned in and connected with their feelings. If it hurts, they won't let you finish and won't want to try it again.

QUICK RELIEF

Five-Minute Tummy Ache Massage for Infants and Children

Mix the essential oil of chamomile into the massage oil. It is a longtime favorite for bellyaches because of its antispasmodic, calming action. Massage the area between the rib cage and the pelvis in long even downward strokes. Then massage the sides of the trunk from under the rib cage to the pelvis in downward strokes. Continue with spiraling clockwise circles around the belly button. Finish with a foot and leg massage to ensure good circulation.

PART IV

Maya Spiritual Illness and Healing

Fortunately for everybody, modern medicine is beginning to catch up with the healing wisdom of the Maya and other ancient cultures. Numerous studies have underlined the link between high blood pressure, arthritis, heart disease, asthma, bronchitis, and even cancer with unresolved emotional stress and distress. At the same time an array of studies in neuroscience is explaining how brain chemistry affects our mental and emotional states. Suddenly—as if it is something new—psychotherapists and medical doctors are once again being taught to consider the importance of the mind-body connection in disease treatment.

"It is folly to ignore the sacred in life or medicine," said Dr. Larry Dossey. "Skirting the spiritual has had a shattering effect on every dimension of contemporary existence."[1]

Centuries ago an ancient Thracian physician said much the same: "You ought not to attempt to cure eyes without head, or head without body, so you should not treat body without soul." The Maya couldn't agree more.

Soul Loss

The Maya recognize diseases of the soul as well as the body and are aware that there are both spiritual and physical *causes* of illness. Underlying their concept of spiritual illness is the concept of loss of ch'ulel, or soul loss.

Soul loss is a universal theme. The Maya, along with other ancient cultures, believe that souls can be frightened away, wander off, or be abducted. Sandra Ingerman has offered more contemporary reasons for soul loss. "Today's soul loss springs from the traumas of modern life," she wrote. "Incest, abuse, loss of a loved one, accidents, wartime experiences, major illness, and surgery are assaults that can catapult the soul from the body. Faced with these kind of stresses, the sensitive human soul may flee the body, never to return."[2]

According to Ingerman, our soul, or a part of our vital essence, separates from us in order to survive the experience by escaping the full impact of pain. "What constitutes trauma varies from one individual to another," she added. "Soul loss can be caused by whatever a person experiences as traumatic, even if another person would not experience it as such."

Children are especially susceptible to soul loss. Their souls are considered to be what Don Elijio called "soft." By this he meant that their souls are not yet strongly connected to the body and are therefore easier to dislodge.

Soul loss leaves people of any age feeling dispirited, weak, fragmented, and disassociated from themselves and the world. Many teenagers and adults make misguided attempts to reconnect with their souls, filling the void with drugs, alcohol, food, or obsessive relationships. Therapy may not help because, as Ingerman said, "nobody's home" to be helped.

Ingerman, trained in both psychotherapy and shamanism, has recommended shamanic journeying in order to reconnect with the lost soul. The ancient tradition of shamanic journeying is the practice of leaving one's body to find a lost soul with the help of spirit guides. It takes years to learn to navigate the spirit world, and it is dangerous for the untrained and uninitiated. Only shamans and their apprentices should attempt the journey.

Like other cultures with shamanic traditions, the Maya have plenty to say about evil spirits that kidnap souls and deposit them in the frightening underworld. Maya shamanic teachings speak of *banditos* who steal souls, and of souls who wait for their owners at the exact spot where they were lost—that is, until an evil spirit comes by and snatches them up. There are Maya shamans who devote themselves to journeying through the dark underworld to retrieve souls.

But as I learned from Don Elijio, the Maya also have safer, gentler ways of luring a lost soul out of the underworld and back into the body. Don Elijio used a complex system of spiritual healing that was just as effective as classic shamanic tools such as drums, rattles, and power animals, sometimes even more so. Many a patient who had been delivered to his doorstep in a desperate state left his clinic under her own steam, lucid and clear-eyed. .

Don Elijio could say prayers into a baby's wrist for fright or cure soul possession. He did not contact the Maya spirits by making the dangerous journey out of ordinary reality. He did his soul work with the help of his sastun, dream visions, prayers, faith, plants, spiritual baths, ritual and ceremony, incense, holy water, and amulets. Faith and prayer were his most powerful healing tools. His spirit guides were the Nine Benevolent Maya Spirits, the Virgin Mary, and a few of his other favorite Catholic saints. He viewed all of his spiritual treatments and rituals as ways of calling the soul back to the body.

Don Elijio also believed that he was balancing the inward and outward flows of a person's energy. The Maya believe that each person has paths of energy coursing in and around the body. That energy, called ch'ulel (the soul or vital life force), is central to health.

The ch'ulel pulsates rhythmically in and out of the body, and the inward and outward flows need to be harmonious and steady. "Not too much, not too little," Don Elijio used to say. When the flow is off balance, too much ch'ulel escapes and the pulsations become chaotic rather than harmonious. The Kekchi Maya consider a spiritual disease to be "the shaking of one's center of balance," according to the anthropologist James Boster, who studied the healing practices of the Kekchi in the 1970s.

Indeed, soul loss knocks a person's entire system out of balance. In traditional Maya healing the healer, as the intermediary between the physical and spiritual worlds, has the ability to focus his or her own ch'ulel on a person in order to help correct the balance between the outward and inward flows.

At the same time the healer replenishes the person's ch'ulel. To accomplish this the healer's ch'ulel combines with the ch'ulel carried by prayer, plants, rituals, incense, and baths. The most powerful form of concentrated ch'ulel is prayer. It is prayer that connects us to the world of the spirits that exists on the other side of the Maya veil. The spirits respond to the prayers by sending ch'ulel back to the person in need. This is true spiritual healing—or healing with spirits.

Physical healing also occurs on a spiritual plane through the transmission of ch'ulel. For example, taking an herbal bath facilitates a ch'ulel exchange between the water, the plants, and the body.

This transmission occurs whether or not a person believes in spirits. As a result, there is some therapeutic value here even for nonbelievers. Of course, believers receive more ch'ulel. Those who believe put up less resistance: energy flows the most freely along paths of least resistance.

Faith

Physical and spiritual healing are more complete and last longer when both the healer and the patient have faith.

Many healers who do this kind of work will first ask you whether you have faith. Don Elijio always asked: "Tiennes fe?" (Do you have faith?) He didn't mind if you didn't have faith in his Maya spirits as long as you had faith in him and a power beyond yourself.

To have faith to heal yourself or others, you need to believe in a god, a goddess, or gods and goddesses, a vague great power that created the earth, or the essence of God within. You also need faith in yourself, the tools you are using, and the knowledge that your prayers will be answered. Remember, some people have faith in the healer—in the scientific or medical degrees on the wall or the healer's personal charisma or ch'ulel level.

The Biology of Ch'ulel

The loss of ch'ulel is a deep internal shock to the entire system at a cellular level that inhibits the immune system, irritates the nervous system, impairs digestion, causes headaches and nightmares, and can mimic serious and chronic diseases like lupus, chronic fatigue syndrome, and rheumatoid arthritis.

The loss of ch'ulel keeps the body trapped in what Dr. Herbert Benson has called the "fight-or-flight" state. Some people live in that state for years and don't know how to escape. Maya spiritual healing is a very effective way to help people escape this vicious circle. It closes down the fight-or-flight reaction and returns us to a more relaxed state of balanced well-being. By reconnecting, recharging, and rebalancing an individual's ch'ulel flow, the

Maya's spiritual healing process changes the chemical makeup of the brain.

It takes the energy of the healer, working with prayers, plants, and spirits, to accomplish this healing. The Maya healer draws on a larger team than the one drawn on by modern medical practitioners, but in the end faith is the energy changer, the catalyst for chemical change.

Do You Have a Spiritual Illness?

Maya healers always begin by assessing whether the origin of an ailment is physical or spiritual. This usually doesn't take a practiced healer very long. She needs only a few moments to check the rhythm and intensity of a person's pulse. In difficult cases, she may need to confer with the spirits to be sure of the origin.

Although the untrained won't be able to use these advanced diagnostic tools, it is possible

Night Terrors and the Spiritually Ill

According to the Maya, night terrors are a primary symptom of many spiritual diseases.

A night terror is more intense than a nightmare. When you awake from a night terror, you sense danger and an eerie presence in the room. You are likely to have heart palpitations.

These occur at night because while asleep the soul's hold on the body is weaker. They can be a sign that soul loss has occurred. A night terror can also be the work of unemployed spirit guides who are angry because the sleeper has not yet awakened to his true calling.

to make a good diagnosis by carefully evaluating the common signs and symptoms. Each of the spiritual illnesses has some of its own unique symptoms, but they all have some in common. Here is a checklist of general symptoms of spiritual illness:

- Nightmares with recurrent themes
- Feeling disconnected from the body
- Feeling depleted and listless
- Bad luck and misfortune
- Frequent domestic quarreling
- A history of substance abuse

- A tendency to be inordinately angry
- Weak immune system
- Sudden bouts of heart palpitations
- A tendency to tearfulness

The Three-Part Treatment for Spiritual Illnesses

The Maya treatments for the four main spiritual illnesses (see page 162) are generally the same. These lovely ch'ulel-enriching rituals will guide you through the healing process.

Please remember that spiritual healing is *not* a science—there are no hard-and-fast rules or formulas. As long as you are sincere, say the prayers with faith and love, and follow your intuition to the best of your ability, you will do fine.

Prayer

A lot of us never learn how to pray, or we associate prayer with stodgy churches and sexist ceremonies. Here are some ways to pray comfortably.

Start by burning some incense. Incense adds power to the ritual of praying and helps to put you in the right frame of mind. Create a little altar for your favorite religious items, icons, sacred objects, and photographs of the people for whom you want to pray. Altars can be a lovely permanent addition to your home.

Then decide to whom or to what you will address your prayers. To tap into healing power you need to have a good relationship with a divine being. This is entirely up to you. It can be the Nine Benevolent Maya Spirits or Jesus, Mohammed, Buddha, Krishna, the Indian gods, or Adonai. Place an image or appropriate reminder of that deity on your altar.

What does matter is that you have a spiritual bank account with this spiritual being. To maintain such an account you need to give love, offerings, service, and prayer to your deity. Furthermore, a practitioner or an individual who uses prayer as part of healing cannot lie, cheat, or steal. Since few of us can meet that criteria at all times, we also need to be able to admit our transgressions and to ask for forgiveness.

If you can't think of your own prayer, here is one Don Elijio taught me. It is a general-purpose prayer, based in part on the Catholic tradition embedded in the Maya world.

In the name of God the Father, God the Son, and God the Holy Spirit. I am the one who prays to the Nine Maya Spirits with my prayer to help sick people. I ask God to help me and I also ask a favor of the Maya spirits that they help me. I believe in them, and I have faith with all my heart in their great power to help and to heal. Nine times I say my prayers. In the name of God the Father, God the Son, and God the Holy Spirit. Amen.

Notice the formula of this simple prayer. It opens with a declaration and invocation to the deity being addressed. It states who you are and what you are asking. It states your faith and closes with a final salutation to the same spiritual power. Using this formula, you can create your own prayers. It is always appropriate to use prayers of your own faith. These prayers should be said with a real depth of meaning, savoring every word and feeling the spiritual energy they create within us. We need not repeat the forced and rushed prayer patterns of our childhood.

If you find you can't pray, ask someone to pray for you. In the Maya world and in other old traditions there are some traditional healers who *only* pray for the sick. These are called *ensalmeros*. *Ensalmo* is "prayer" in Spanish. These prayer-makers are able to concentrate their energy and focus healing intent on a patient, while at the same time asking their spirit guides for assistance. Some patients have related that, when they received healing prayers, they experienced a physical sensation of tremendous energy, a force that could be described as a strong, pushing wind passing through the body.

You may not be able to find an ensalmero, but you can ask a religious leader—a rabbi, priest, or other minister—or a layperson of abiding faith who prays well, or just a friend to pray for you. You can also go to a religious service and pray along with other people.

Maya healing prayers are thought to be most powerful when offered on Thursdays or Fridays. The source of this custom is obscure, but instructions for its practice have been handed down through generations. Don Elijio gave one explanation: these are the days when the Nine Benevolent Maya Spirits are believed to wander the earth to answer the prayers of the faithful. However, healers pray seven days a week for their patients with good results. Don Elijio always set aside time on Thursday or Friday to send some special prayers to the Maya spirits in order to keep his spiritual account full.

Herbal Baths

Plants are good ch'ulel carriers and work well for herbal baths prepared for spiritual healing. You can use rue, basil, marigold, rosemary, red and white roses, motherwort, Saint-John's-wort, or sage. My favorites are rue, basil, and marigold, but when they are not available, I have used all of the others with great success. You can use one or more plants to make your bath.

It is important to decide on the number of plants, flowers, or branches to gather. Numbers are powerful purveyors of ch'ulel. Some healers like to gather four branches, four plants, or four flowers of different herbs. Some use nine and others seven.

I fluctuate between four and nine, depending on how much I think any plant can give without being stressed. So I might gather four sprigs of rue, nine flowering branches of marigold, and nine branches of basil. This is not an exact science, and there are really no specific formulas. Intuition and spontaneity play a role when gathering herbs for spiritual healing.

Also, remember not to mistreat or stress any plants by overharvesting or pulling too roughly on their leaves or stems. Imagine if you went up to a person, grabbed him by the collar, and pulled him roughly, demanding that he come to help you. You wouldn't get very far, would you? We need to be just as thoughtful and polite to plants in order to get them to help us. The plants, like us, say the Maya, are spiritual beings in physical bodies.

Don't forget to give the prayer of faith and thanks to the plant so that the spirit of the plant follows you home to help with the healing.

Here are some sample herbal baths for spiritual healing:

A Summer Bath with Fresh Plants

9 sprigs rue, about 6 inches long
9 branches marigold, with flowers about 12 inches long
4 branches basil, about 12 inches long
   or:
4 branches motherwort, about 12 inches long
9 branches sage, about 12 inches long
9 branches Saint-John's-wort, about 12 inches long

Fill a washtub or your largest pot with water. Place the plants in the water and squeeze them between your hands. This is another good time to pray for what you wish to accomplish with this bath. Do what feels right and comes from the heart.

Breathe deeply and gratefully of the aroma, for this too is healing. After ten minutes or so, when the plants are well crushed and the water has taken on color and aroma, set it aside for one to eight hours. You can make this preparation in the morning and bathe that night, or you can prepare in the evening and bathe in the morning.

If you have a bathtub, fill it half full with tap water at a temperature of your liking. Then scoop a half-cup of the herbal water out of the pot and drink it. Pour the remainder of the herbal water into the tub.

You can strain out the leaves and flowers first if you wish to make cleaning up easier, but it is lovely to bathe surrounded by floating flowers and leaves. Some people pour all the plants into the tub and gather them up in their hands to rub onto their face and body.

Soak thirty minutes, relaxing and meditating on the purpose of the bath. Burn copal incense. This is a good time to pray.

If you have no bathtub, carry the pot of herbs into the shower. Sit on a stool or chair in the shower and with a bowl slowly pour the herbal water over your body. You can add some hot tap water to the pot of herbs for a warmer bath. It's best to put a strainer of some kind in the drain to avoid clogging.

If at all possible, don't towel-dry. Let your body air-dry to retain the goodness of the herbs as much as possible.

A Winter Bath with Dried Plants

If fresh herbs are not available, you need one cup of a dried herb or a combination of herbs for each gallon of water. Boil in a large pot for five minutes. Steep for an hour. Use as for a summer bath. Here's a suggestion for a nice winter bath.

$\frac{1}{4}$ c dried rosemary
$\frac{1}{4}$ c dried sage
$\frac{1}{4}$ c dried roses
$\frac{1}{4}$ c dried rue

Incense

The Maya favor copal resin and dried rosemary leaves for treatment of all spiritual ailments. You can find out how to order these in the Resources appendix, or you can use dried sage leaves or cedar.

To burn incense you need charcoal. Small round pieces of easy-to-light charcoal are now sold in most stores that feature incense (see Resources appendix).

If you have a fireplace, scoop out a hot coal and place it in a fireproof container that can be placed in another object so that you can move it around the house. I use my old Chinese wok—I can easily grasp the wooden handle without getting burned. You can also purchase an incense burner.

Burn the incense while bathing and either before or after the bath. Carry it around the house into every room. This is another good time to pray.

The Spiritual Diseases of the Maya

The Maya speak of four major kinds of spiritual illnesses: *susto* or fright, *pesar* or grief, *tristeza* or sadness, and *invidia* or envy.

It is unlikely that the words *tristeza, invidia, susto,* and *pesar* will pop into our modern minds when we are down or afraid. We are more likely to say, "Ahh, my heart is broken, I'm grieving for a loved one, I feel empty and disconnected." But within these Maya categories of spiritual illness fall such basic human experiences as depression, feelings of worthlessness and despair, feeling unlucky, recurrent nightmares, and post-traumatic stress.

Susto—Fright

The most common spiritual disease of the Maya is *susto*, which means "fright" and usually refers to a trauma or shock.

Susto is one of the manifestations of soul loss. The soul is thought to be frightened out of the body by some traumatic event. Some scholars think the concept of susto came from the Spaniards. Others say that the concept of soul loss was native to the Maya before the arrival of the Spaniards.

Susto can happen to adults, children, and infants. Children and infants are especially vulnerable because they have less ch'ulel and a weaker hold on their souls. People suffering from susto are often not aware of it and as a result can go through life with a variety of undiagnosable diseases.

As Don Elijio liked to tell his patients who claimed to have been to several medical clinics in search of a cure, "La maquina no muestra" (The machine doesn't show it).

Susto affects the emotional, spiritual, and physical equilibrium. Fright is a great thief of ch'ulel and sends a deep internal shock through the entire system. That shock inhibits the immune system from fighting off disease, irritates the nervous system, haunts the psyche, disturbs digestion, and causes headaches, nightmares, and panic attacks. Some people have the feeling that "nothing is right" in their lives. Others have strange diagnoses from medical clinics like "some kind of leukemia," a previously unknown type of stress-related disorder, or no diagnosis at all.

How Do You Know If You Have Susto? Here are some guidelines to consider.

Adults If the traumatic event was recent, susto sufferers may feel a sudden disruption in their emotional balance. If the event that caused susto occurred in childhood, they may have a long history of vague illness, failed romance, fears, and depression. Susto sufferers are easily frightened and jumpy. They often break into tears without warning and feel confused. They may be anxious, have heart palpitations, and exhibit antisocial behavior. Other symptoms may include falling-out hair, dry skin, rashes, and eating pattern disturbances. Indigestion and diarrhea often alternate with constipation.

Events That Can Cause Susto

The kinds of things that can lead to susto are common to people all over the world. No one escapes susto entirely. Whenever I explain the concept of susto in my lectures and ask how many people can relate, invariably every person in the room raises a hand. Of course, what may cause susto in one person may go right by another.

   Some events that cause serious cases in children are

Witnessing a frightening event of any kind
Seeing a violent fight erupt between adults in the household
Going to a wake or funeral too early in life
The sudden death or suicide of a family member
Violent spanking and physical abuse
Violent potty training
Sexual abuse and incest
Violent movies and television programs
Being in an accident involving a car, bus, airplane, or train
Fires, hurricanes, tornadoes, floods, explosions
Abandonment
Severe bullying by peers

Being awakened from a peaceful nap by a frightening noise and experiencing a fall or minor injury are the kind of events that cause less serious, "temporary" susto.

   In adults, events that could cause long-term or temporary susto are

Witnessing an accident in which another is injured
Being in a serious accident
Nearly being involved in an accident
Rape, incest, sexual abuse
Domestic violence
Being in a car, airplane, boat, or train crash
Witnessing a murder or violent death
The suicide of a friend or family member
Being mugged or being present at a robbery
Witnessing fires, explosions, or shootings
Natural disasters such as earthquakes, hurricanes, tornadoes, and floods
War and its consequent events
Receiving sudden bad news

Infants Susto babies are cranky and unhappy. These little ones do not play or smile as much as they should and may try to slap their caregivers. They certainly do not sleep well. These are the babies who take an hour to fall asleep and then wake up howling in ten minutes. They don't eat well and throw up frequently. Their stools may turn a greenish color, and their urine may have a strong smell. Rashes and diarrhea are common.

Children The child with susto behaves poorly and erratically and probably gets into trouble at school. There seems to be no pattern to his behavior: it is hard to determine what will make the child cry or throw a tantrum. These children have trouble making friends, and when they do have playmates, they often fuss more than play. Many do not even know how to play and may be labeled hyperactive or emotionally disturbed. They have erratic sleep patterns and night terrors about monsters and scary creatures. Nervous twitches, finger biting or sucking, and rocking are common. As teenagers, these kids are more likely than others to exhibit antisocial behavior, fall into bad company, and experiment with drugs and alcohol in search of relief.

A Lifetime of Susto: A Case from Ukraine A few years ago, at a conference, I gave a talk on Maya spiritual healing. Afterward a woman in her fifties came up to me and asked for some time to talk about her illness. She was pale and thin and spoke with an almost inaudible voice that seemed not to get enough air from her lungs. I had to listen very carefully in order to hear her. She explained that she had been diagnosed with "some kind of leukemia" and had been ill for many decades with little hope of a cure.

I felt her pulse and immediately recognized that there had been a great fright in her life, probably a very long time ago. A person with susto has a pulse that is very rapid and jumpy. When I asked her whether any traumatic events had occurred in her life, the woman began to cry.

She told me a horrifying story about growing up in Communist Ukraine during a time of great political and social upheaval. Her parents were political activists, and one day Communist Party officials burst into their home and murdered her parents before her eyes. She was sent to an orphanage where she was bullied and sexually abused. It was clear that she had never recovered from these physical and emotional traumas. Through her tears she told me that her life felt empty and devoid of purpose and meaning. She found solace only in gardening and playing the piano.

I said the nine Maya prayers for susto for her three times over that weekend and gave her some copal incense to burn at home every day. I instructed her to take an herbal bath twice weekly with rue, basil, and marigold. As a devoted gardener, she had all three of them growing in her backyard.

This is an excerpt from the letter I received from her three months later:

> I am writing to give you an update on what has happened since I saw you and you diagnosed me with susto. Since then, only good things have occurred to me. My blood condition has improved, and so has my overall physical, mental, and emotional health. I feel like my soul has returned to me, thus feeling whole. I am aware that I must continue doing the prayers and remedies you prescribed for nine months, and I will. The change in my health has been gradual and sure. Within a month my desire to live began to return, and now I am feeling better than I have in thirty years. Taking the herbal baths and burning the copal became a beacon of strength and hope for me

Healing Susto Can Help Your Marriage and Your Sex Life

Many people who have experienced sexual abuse, rape, or incest can benefit from susto treatment, which helps them to go beyond previous physical and emotional limits. It has helped couples get pregnant, rekindle intimacy, and gain a deeper understanding of each other.

A Maya woman came to see me with her husband. She was shy and sat silently while her husband related this story to me.

"My wife's life is not right," he told me. "She is not the same person I married two years ago. She has stopped cooking. She does not clean the house. I have been patient, I think, but now believe that there is something wrong that no doctor can cure. She has stomachaches, bad dreams, and sometimes cries for no reason.

"I think this all started when we went to visit my brothers who own a ranch in another country. We spent a few days on the beach, and while there she decided to take a walk on the beach by herself. I didn't like the idea, but she went anyway by herself. While out on her walk, a man ran out of the bushes and grabbed her from behind. He pulled off her waist bag containing her money and hit her several times on the face and head. He might have done more, but she screamed and someone came running to help. The man escaped, and we were never able to find him or the purse again. Do you think she has a bad case of susto?"

Central American people are very familiar with susto and its effects but often do not know how to treat it. I took her pulse and found it rapid and bouncing. It was evident that the woman had very bad susto.

I said the Maya prayers for her nine times. Then I went into my healing garden and picked some basil, marigold, and rue. When I returned, she was talking excitedly with her husband. He looked at me and nodded in approval as if to say, "The healing has already begun."

For good measure, I repeated the nine prayers, this time with a small branch of each of the three plants placed in a cross formation over her pulses and forehead. This adds a great deal of ch'ulel to the prayer.

I gave her copal incense to burn at home on Friday and told her to take an herbal bath. She was to repeat the incense burning and herbal bathing for three Fridays consecutively.

A month later she wrote me a very sweet letter saying that she was finally able to put the mugging incident behind her and was feeling a lot better. She was engaged once again in her household, enjoying a good relationship with her husband, and no longer plagued by bad dreams.

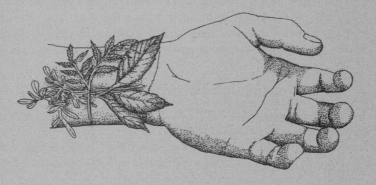

because after every bath I felt better and better. It was as though my trouble and sickness were washed away. My doctors say that my blood count and white cells have returned to normal. I feel renewed and like I have just been let out of jail after a life sentence.

Susto in Utero: A Case from Belize   In Belize a young mother came to see me about her three-month-old infant, who would not sleep more than a few minutes during the day and woke up every hour at night. He was not gaining weight properly and was so cranky that she felt she could not cope.

When I felt the baby boy's pulse, the diagnosis of susto was easy. She told me that when she was seven months pregnant, there was a terrible fire where she worked that had destroyed two buildings.

"We had to fight that fire for two hours with hoses and buckets," she cried. "We were all in danger of serious injury, and I was terribly frightened."

Her baby in the womb, affected by her experience, was now exhibiting classic susto symptoms. Both mother and baby had to be treated with prayers, herbal baths, and copal incense. I said the appropriate Maya prayers into their pulses that day, and together we went to my garden and gathered enough rue, basil, and marigold to bathe them both three times during the next week. She was to burn copal in her house every day for nine days.

A short time later the woman told me that her baby now slept for two hours in the morning and the afternoon, went to sleep at 7:00 P.M., and woke up only once during the night for a breast-feeding. He was playful, happy, and starting to gain weight— "gordo y contento" (fat and happy), said the mother.

Here is a special prayer for susto:

In the name of God the Father, God the Son, and God the Holy Spirit, I am the one who prays for susto. I ask God to help me, and I ask the Nine Maya Spirits to help me too. I say these prayers nine times to release this susto from the flesh of ————. I have faith with all my heart that this prayer, these herbs, baths, and incense, will cure the susto of ————. In the name of God the Father, God the Son, and God the Holy Spirit.

Repeat this prayer nine times—three times each while holding the right and left pulse at each wrist, and three while holding both hands over the head.

Tristeza—Sadness

This spiritual disease includes many of those nebulous states of darkness that modern folk lump under one word—depression. Don Elijio called tristeza sufferers the "I don't want to do anything and I don't care about anything" folks. Their zest for life has gone, and their courage to carry on is weak. They give up readily and feel that life is unfair to them and that nothing ever has and never will go right for them. They are often pale, and because they either don't eat enough or eat too much, they lose or gain excessive amounts of weight.

Tristeza can be accompanied by anger, resentment, and an uncontrollable urge to rehash hurtful events. At other times tristeza sufferers can give no reason for their feelings of hopelessness. The emotions of people with tristeza are like a runaway horse and cart. Obsessed with their misfortunes, they are like dark clouds, and they wear down the patience of friends. Indeed, they lose friends.

ANCIENT WISDOM
Special Treatments for Tristeza

An old-time favorite of the Mexican Maya is to take nine white flowers of the same variety—nine white roses, nine white hibiscus—to the river or a creek at noon. The tristeza sufferer throws the flowers into the current one by one and watches them intently as they float away.

Another cure is to take a new calabash gourd bowl to the river at noon. Scoop out a bit of river water and take nine sips while saying nine "Our Fathers." The remaining water in the calabash should be thrown over the shoulder back into the river.

Others swear that tristeza—especially the broken heart variety—can be cured by eating handfuls of unshelled pumpkin seeds.

The person with tristeza is like a battery that has gradually run down. Sadness is a powerful ch'ulel sapper. Unlike a shock that violently sucks out ch'ulel, tristeza is like a slow leak that if unchecked can lead to that familiar feeling of emptiness.

Years of Tristeza: A Case from New York A filmmaker living in Manhattan came to see me while on vacation in Belize. He was frail and pale with a stooped posture and tentative bearing. "I've been in therapy for depression now for ten years," he told me. "I can't really say that it helps very much. I thought perhaps it would be worth a try to come and see you." We talked for a while, and it was true that there was no overt cause in the past or present for his long-term bouts with depression. He wasn't clear on why he felt the way he did, and I wasn't either. So I thought our best solution would be to do just what we do for all spiritual ailments, regardless of cause: prayers, baths, and incense. I said the Maya prayers for him, then taught him to make the herbal baths and to burn copal. He wrote back a few months later saying that while he certainly was not cured, he did feel as though a heavy emotional burden was slowly lifting and that for the first time in years he felt hopeful that he might get better.

Treatment for Severe Cases For severe, chronic cases of tristeza, here's what to do. For some, this simple treatment can be more trans-formative than years of psychotherapy. The person feels as if a great cloud of heavy darkness has been lifted and he can begin to live again.

Say nine prayers into the person's pulses—three at the right radial pulse, three at the left radial pulse, and three over the fore-head. If doing this for yourself, say the nine prayers out loud with reverence.

Take baths with rue and basil.

Place a rue sprig under the tongue, sucking on the leaves and swallowing the juices for twenty-four hours. Each sprig of rue will require about an hour to consume and should then be replaced. Before you put a sprig in your mouth, test whether you are allergic to it by pulling off a tiny leaf and rubbing it on the skin of the inside of your elbow. If you are allergic, you will have a red, itchy reaction within twenty minutes. If you are allergic, pregnant, or can't find rue, use basil.

I like to suggest to patients that they purchase a rue plant from a nursery and keep it in their home, caring for it lovingly, praying for grace from the "herb of grace" (one of rue's common names) and meditating with the plant in order to communicate their needs for healing.

Burning copal or rosemary incense in the home should also be done for at least three consecutive days.

Invidia—Envy

While we do think about fear and depression, the concept of envy, or *invidia* as it is called in Spanish, doesn't merit much thought in modern life. The idea of envy lives more in a religious dimension than in modern psychology. Envy is a largely unspoken reality in our culture. This is not so for the Maya. Their analysis of envy can provide a valuable dimension to understanding human interaction.

Since I grew up in a religious immigrant household, I heard about envy every day. My mother's family was from Iran (Persia back then), and my father was born in Italy. Both the Mediterranean and the Middle Eastern cultures are conscious of the concept of envy.

We children were raised as Catholics. In those days children had to wear a red scapula around their necks to proclaim their faith. My Italian grandmother Isola always placed a clove of garlic inside my scapula to protect me from envy. Penna, my Persian grandmother, gave me a silver hand from Persia to place over the garlic clove.

Grandma Isola told us that envy is natural and that all human beings experience it from time to time. That is why, she said, it is wise to protect yourself with garlic and lucky charms such as silver hands, eyes, and horns. She said that envy toward another is a dangerous weapon that can make another very ill, so her advice was to say this little ditty: "I wish I was as pretty as she is and she was even prettier." Or: "I wish I had a house as lovely as hers and she had a nicer house."

So the Maya concept of envy wasn't foreign to me. I did not immediately dismiss it as superstition. According to Don Elijio and other Maya healers, "envy is the Maya's national disease," and I would have plenty of opportunities to observe the devastating effects that envy can have on human life. Although neglected, the concept of envy is part of our universal subconsciousness. Pre-Judeo-Christian pagans and early Jews also believed that envy could cause physical harm.

How Envy Works As a spiritual disease, envy develops when you are subjected daily to a regular current of negativity—through thought or deed—projected by a person who feels envy or jealousy; it can provoke both physical and emotional problems. The barrage of negative energy saps ch'ulel. Envy is an attempt to steal ch'ulel from coworkers, relatives, employees, maids, friends, and acquaintances. We can be the object of envy or the perpetrator of envy.

"Maybe you eat well, live in a nice house, have a good job and beautiful children," Don Elijio used to tell his patients. "Every day your coworker or neighbor looks upon you with envy and jealousy. Soon it makes you sick." As the Maya see it, success, good fortune, good looks, happiness, fame, wealth, romance, and children can all breed envy in others. Often it is no fault of the object of envy. I have an image of envy streaming forth like a river of sludge, darkening and drowning all in its wake.

Envy is not always bad. On the positive side, envy can make us improve ourselves if we are smart enough to use another's good fortune as a model. This person looks upon another's good fortune and says: "Hmm, I could do that. Step aside and watch me do even better." He or she is using envy as a stepping-stone, becoming motivated to take action and improve productivity. This kind of envy is fleeting and inspirational and does not hurt anyone.

Envy that buys into the concept of "limited good" is harmful. If you believe that there is only so much good to go around and your neighbor has more than you think is his fair share, you are bound to think that there is less available for you. This erroneous belief comes from the fear of not having enough. It assumes that you know what is the right amount of goodness and bounty for your neighbor.

Are You Suffering from Envy? If the jealousy is coming from a person in or close to your home, you may feel convinced that you will find happiness again only if you move. When the envy streams forth from a coworker, you'll feel that you must change jobs or professions to find contentment. If the jealousy is coming from a coworker, you will feel much better when you leave work. If it is streaming from a neighbor or someone in your household, you will feel confused and depressed while at home, but better when you leave.

You may feel a lack of interest in the daily affairs of life. Your burning desires and interests may seem boring and unworthy of effort. You may sleep poorly, lack appetite, experience nightmares, have stomach problems, and lose self-confidence. You may have a feeling of foreboding and lack any sense of peace or harmony.

Another symptom of envy is bad luck or feeling down on your luck. You may feel that you are always in the wrong place at the wrong time and that life is a struggle on every level.

How We Invite Envy We can unintentionally invite envy by our own sense of superiority, criticism, and disdain of others. Malicious gossiping, boasting, and unfriendliness are surefire ways to attract envy. Pain is the arrow that transmits envy. So keep a quiet counsel to avoid the arrows of envy. It may still happen, but at least you'll know that you were not the agent of your own misfortune. An old Creole proverb of Belize says, "Self-praise is no praise at all."

Some kinds of gossip can cause and send envy. Gossip that belittles and criticizes another person so that we can feel better about ourselves is what leads to trouble. This is the kind of exchange that usually leaves us feeling worse afterward, not better. It's not the same as constructive discussion in which we talk to a friend in order to vent stored-up emotions about another friend, analyzing the situation as we verbally walk through it again. Any gossip should end with a blessing such as, "Well, God bless her."

Amulets Unfortunately, you can be cured of envy by a healer only to have it recur over and over again if the one who envies remains

ANCIENT WISDOM

Special Treatments for Envy

Treatment for envy is much like treatment for the other spiritual diseases—prayer, herbal baths, incense, and teas. The prayers, baths, and burning of incense need to be repeated at least once weekly. Beneficial teas are rosemary, basil, and rue.

However, envy can be very stubborn to dislodge, and it is sometimes necessary to get professional help to dispel the negativity. Receiving a blessing from a priest, rabbi, priestess, or minister is also very helpful. Reading spiritual literature regularly can help. These are all ways to replace lost ch'ulel.

in regular contact with you. As a result, the Maya wear protective amulets that repel the currents of negative ch'ulel. The amulets are prepared in a specified manner with certain natural objects and then blessed with ancient and sacred prayers that ask the Maya spirits for protection, help, and blessings. These can be secured only from a h'men because they require the blessing of a sastun.

What to Do If You Feel Envious Envy is natural to all humans. Each of us will send envy and experience envy at different times. Once a dear friend and I went to visit another friend who had just purchased a new home and invited us over to have a look.

The house, a quaint old Victorian beauty with a spacious front porch, was enormous and had been lovingly remodeled. On the way home my friend admitted that she felt jealous of her friend's good fortune and was ashamed of her feelings. I shared my Grandma Isola's solution, and together we said, "I wish I had a house as beautiful as Mary's, and I wish she had an even better one." I have used Grandma Isola's advice many times.

If you recognize that you are jealous and make up your mind to do something about it, you are already on the path to healing. Perform this ritual: place rue under your tongue and say, "I am now free of envy and jealousy, and I wish Tom and Mary good fortune in their lives. I too can achieve, succeed, and excel." Then take an herbal bath and burn copal or another powerful incense such as sage, cedar, or rosemary in your home.

ANCIENT WISDOM

Sweeping Away Misfortune

The Maya sweep the stairs and the entranceway to their homes with a broom dipped in a bucket filled with water in which basil leaves have been squeezed and steeped. They do this to ward off envy and also when they are feeling down on their luck.

Perform the basil-water sweep for nine consecutive days, starting on a Thursday or a Friday. Basil water can also be sprinkled all around the house, especially where you sleep, eat, and rest. While sprinkling the water, say out loud: "All bad luck must now leave me and this place. I have faith with all my heart that this sacred water and these prayers will dispel all misfortune and change my life for the better."

Cleansing a House of Envy You never know what kind of negative feelings have been left in a house after a divorce, argument, robbery, or some other stressful event. Buildings, objects, even plants can be the recipient of negative ch'ulel.

My friend Louise, who is a single mother, had employed an El Salvadoran housekeeper for two and a half years. Elsa, the housekeeper, was older than Louise, and once she felt comfortable in the job she became bossy and belligerent.

She thought she was a better mother than Louise and often let her know it. She always let the children know that she was a better cook and a better companion, and that she loved them as much, if not more, than their mother.

Elsa was particularly possessive over one ailing poinsettia plant that Louise had had for several years. She nursed it back to health and kept it in the kitchen next to the sink. Elsa often brought Louise over to the plant and said, "I saved it when you couldn't."

> ### For Catholics
>
> Don Elijio always thought that holy water from the Catholic Church had special power. He had a bottle of holy water ready and at hand in his little doctor's bag and used it daily for spiritual healing. Holy water can be obtained from a font in any Catholic church and stored in glass bottles (not plastic) for up to a year. Mash a sprig of rue into a quarter-cup of the holy water and drink. Place nine drops of holy water in tea for healing. I like to add a capful to the water whenever I bathe or bless a house.

Louise didn't like Elsa's behavior but had no stomach for firing her. She kept quiet until Elsa started keeping erratic hours and got into the habit of yelling at her in front of others. When she brought this up, Elsa hit the roof. She ran out of the house, then came back later when no one was home. She threw the dirty laundry all over the living room floor and then came back no more.

After all this, Louise asked me to cleanse her house. We did it together, using the following ritual. Afterward a great sense of peace came over the household.

Within six hours the healthy poinsettia plant, sitting beside the sink, shriveled up and died.

The Evil Eye

Evil eye, or *mal ojo*, though related to envy, is more acute and less intentional.

One can become the victim of the evil eye in various ways. If you wear an outfit that looks absolutely wonderful and someone looks upon you with intense envy and even hatred, that glance can make you feel depressed or ill. The same goes for someone who has just won a prize or trophy, bought a new home, or earned a promotion.

Maya people believe that gazing upon a newborn baby with thoughts of envy can make the infant ill. Thus the Maya custom of covering the face of infants with a light cloth to protect them from "hot eyes" or "bad eyes."

Everybody knows somebody who has an intense stare or glare that makes us uncomfortable at times. People with hot eyes need to be aware of their impact. One Maya healer told me of a neighbor who always sent word ahead with a child when she was to arrive for a visit so that the parrot's cage could be covered in order to protect the bird from her hot eye.

Symptoms of the evil eye can be sore weepy eyes, with pus or phlegm, sudden appearance of hot, itchy skin rash, sleep disturbances with nightmares, disinterest in the usual affairs of daily life, and an inability to get along with loved ones or family members.

The treatment is the same as for envy.

Many Christians believe in the evil eye. And according to Miriam Chaiken, early Jews thought the evil eye was a demon. "A person could without knowing it, possess an evil eye. The glare of such a person was believed to bring misfortune, as was that of a jealous person." The Jews used amulets, spitting, the number three, and other tools to ward off the evil eye.

Cleansing a house of envy is easy to do and an extremely healing ritual. It moves the negative energy out of the walls, carpets, clothing, and everything else inside the house. For the ritual to work, you must have faith in yourself and faith in the plants and healing tools at your disposal.

Always remember that when doing this work for yourself or others you must never show off—*never*. Be quiet and humble. Bragging is most inadvisable. The less said the better. Talking about this spiritual healing work weakens the effects.

Also, do not do this in the presence of a lot of people. One on one is the best. Family members may be present together. Skeptics and nonbelievers will weaken the beginner, and it is advisable not to have them present.

Begin with prayer—to the particular spirit with whom you have established that special spiritual relationship of give-and-take (not just take). Burn incense throughout the house. Carry it from room to room saying your prayers with faith, gratitude, and love. Give each person a sprig of rue under the tongue and squeeze some rue, basil, and marigold into water.

Let the plants sit in the water for a few minutes in sunlight if possible while you carry the incense about. Then, with your hands or with a few tied-up branches of marigold and basil, sprinkle the plant water all around the house while praying to have envy and jealousy dispelled from the house because they are doing harm.

Sprinkle with abandon into the closets, pantries, bathrooms, showers, under the beds and desks, and pay special attention to the four corners of the house. Sprinkle water over the inhabitants of the house as well.

If you can do this on a Thursday or Friday, so much the better, but if that is not possible, so be it. Your faith alone will balance the disadvantage of the day of the week.

This cleansing has a tremendous beneficial effect on the entire household. There is a palpable difference afterward—the home feels light and peaceful. Hope and clarity reign.

Pesar—Grief

Grief is another emotion common to all humanity. No one escapes bouts of grief, which by nature depletes our reserves of ch'ulel. Grief is necessary to overcome our sadness over the loss of a loved one through death. It is also a natural result of a romantic loss, a divorce, and other major unwelcome changes in life. The grief of children over being moved from one place to another can last for years—even a lifetime.

Do You Have Pesar? The most common symptom of this ailment is deep, mournful sighs that seem to come from the depths of the soul. The person's normal pattern of breathing is shallow, as though the emotional pain is in the chest and any movement from there hurts. Symptoms in children include tearfulness, crankiness, sleeplessness, inability to play, and general malaise.

Grief often comes hand in hand with fright, especially among people who have lost a loved one to a violent, sudden death such as a murder, suicide, or crash. The sufferer is haunted by memories of the deceased and tortured by mental images of their last, final moments. Sometimes even talking to a counselor and sharing the pain is not enough to dispel the horror from their lives.

The treatment for pesar is prayer, bathing, and burning incense.

Pent-up Pesar: A Case from Canada A young Canadian woman came to see me in my clinic in Belize. She had moved to Belize a few years before to start an organic farm. Three months earlier her younger brother—with whom she was very close—was killed in a car accident on his way to the airport to catch a flight to visit her for the first time in her new home.

The woman had the following symptoms: swollen lymph glands, a bladder infection, insomnia, indigestion, loose bowels, fatigue, depression, and a sense of impending doom that she could not shake. She had been to a medical clinic for tests and been told that, besides her bladder infection, everything was normal.

She told me that when she first heard of her brother's death, she felt a great stab of pain in her abdomen that had never completely gone away.

"It's as though I have an icy knot in my guts," she told me. "My appetite is completely gone. I've lost thirty-five pounds since he died. I loved my brother dearly and completely. We were best friends as well as siblings. We dated together as teenagers, bonded as a unit against our parents, and each of us was a source of support and inspiration for the other. We talked on the phone regularly, and I was so excited about his first visit to see me in Belize. It seems that I can't shake my grief and I can't stop thinking about him in that car, the crash, and what he must have felt. I guess I'm haunted. I used to have a very active dream life and looked forward to going to sleep. My dreams are recorded in a special notebook. Since my brother died, I have not remembered a single dream."

I went out to my rue plant and pulled off a few branches after saying the plant prayer. I returned to the clinic and placed a tiny piece of a branch under her tongue and used the other two sprigs to form a cross over her pulses and said a prayer for grief.

Almost immediately the dam of tears opened and flowed and flowed. She sobbed uncontrollably, and it was good. I prepared a bath for her right then and there and bathed her myself with rue, basil, and marigold while she sat naked in the sun on my verandah. Moment by moment we could both feel the fright and the grief clearing from her body, mind, and soul.

I burned copal under her and around her and said the prayers for pesar again after the bath. Then she lay down for a nap in the clinic, and there she stayed in peaceful repose for three hours.

When she awoke, she said she had dreamed about her brother. He was in a good place, and he told her to be at peace because he was happy and fine. "I'm still on vacation," he told her in the dream, "and I haven't yet figured out what my work here will be."

Since that day this woman has been well and productive. The knot in her stomach is gone, she can eat again, her color is back, her hair is full and shiny. She enjoyed the herbal bath so much that she started growing rue, basil, and marigold and bathes herself regularly. She reports that her dreams are more vivid on those days.

Best of all, she rarely thinks of her brother's violent death. Instead, she remembers their good times together and gives thanks for his life while he was with her and their parents.

Broken Hearts   Broken hearts are so common, yet so few know how to help themselves gracefully pass through the pain and grief. The Maya recognize that the broken heart is a spiritual disease expressed through physical symptoms, including sleeplessness, anxiety, uncontrollable thoughts, eating disorders, loss or gain of weight, confusion, difficulty with decisionmaking, and general depression.

Here's a story with a happy ending about one brokenhearted woman.

A young American pharmacy student was attending a student seminar at Ix Chel Farm. During the lecture on Maya spiritual healing I could see that she was greatly troubled. She approached me after class and asked whether she could speak to me in private.

"It's as though you were talking right to me the whole time," she told me. "Just a week before we came on this trip my boyfriend broke up with me, and it totally devastated me. I have not stopped crying the entire time. He is here right now and is having a romance with one of the other girls on this trip. I am mortified, humiliated, sad, brokenhearted, and I feel as though I am being tortured every minute of the day. Can you help me? Is there anything in Maya medicine for me?"

"As a matter of fact, there is," I told her. "Follow me." I took her by the hand and led her to the nursery where my beloved rue plants grow. Rue is my personal plant ally who has helped me so much. I sat before the plants for a moment and said the prayer of faith and thanksgiving. I also mentioned the student's name and asked rue to help her over this difficult time. Then I pinched off a sprig about three inches in length and told her to put a tiny piece of it under her tongue. I told her to suck on it and swallow the juices, then to replace it with another tiny piece three times until she went to bed.

The following morning at around 7:30 A.M. she was the first student to appear. She found me working in the plant nursery.

I had to laugh when she declared with such force and power, "You know what, Dr. Arvigo? I've decided that he did me a favor!"

She was right!

What can you do for a broken heart?

Prayers First and foremost, the sufferer requires a major boost by repeating healing prayers that address the grief and sense of loss. If praying for someone else, say the prayers while placing both your hands on the top of the person's head. If saying them for yourself, kneel or sit in front of a lit green candle. Say the prayers every day for nine consecutive days. Blow out the candle after each prayer session and relight it for the next. On the ninth day let the candle burn down.

Herbal Bath Follow the directions for preparing an herbal bath on page 59. There are so many good plants—fresh or dry—to choose from for a broken heart: marigold, basil, rosemary, oregano, thyme, sage, cedar, melissa, queen of the meadow, motherwort, chamomile, linden flower, lavender, rose geranium, lemon verbena. If you have several of them in the garden, sit with the plants for a moment or two silently explaining what your need is—to overcome the sense of loss, the rejection, the loss of dreams for the future, whatever, and wait to see which plants call your attention the most. It may be one, two, three, or four plants. If you can locate only one or two, no problem—that will be fine. Use what you have available to you with faith and confidence, and the results will speak for themselves.

> ANCIENT WISDOM
>
> Another Way to Banish Pesar
>
> The Maya eat roasted or raw pumpkin seeds by the handful daily until the sadness and grief go away.

Meditate while you squeeze the plants into the water with your bare hands. Think about your wishes for the future and what you would like to come out of this bath ritual—for instance, a fresh start and freedom from painful memories and sadness.

The bath itself is a good time for positive affirmations such as

"With this sacred water, I wash away all sadness and begin to live wholly again."
"I have faith with all my heart that this bath and these prayers will relieve me completely."

Repeat the bath every three days, at least three times, even if you feel wonderful after the first bath.

Herbs to Drink For the broken heart, the Maya always choose fresh rue stems and leaves. Sit silently with the rue plant and explain your need. Pinch off a tiny end of one of the branches—about one inch—and place it under your tongue to suck on gradually while swallowing the juice. Repeat this once or twice daily—three times daily if you are in the worst part of the breakup.

If you are allergic to rue, try Saint-John's-wort. It's a wonderful herb and easy to find as a hot tea, a capsule, or a tincture. Do not take Saint-John's-wort or rue if you are pregnant. In that case a pinch of either rosemary or basil is a good substitute.

Incense Allow the smoke to engulf you while you pray, bathe, sip tea, or chew on your leaves. Burn this incense in the room where you and your lover slept or lived. The purpose of the incense is to remove the emotional and spiritual "leftovers" from the air in the house and its rooms. Carry the incense to wherever you are flooded with memories from the relationship, remembering to concentrate and focus your mind on what changes you are trying to accomplish with this exercise. This is also a good time to pray and to state your faith as well.

Death of a Loved One This spiritual illness is an aspect of pesar or grief. It is different from the grief of the broken heart because of its finality.

Grief over the death of a loved one is a natural, necessary process that no one can or should try to escape. A normal amount of grief honors and praises the life of that special person and acknowledges that there will forever be an empty space that was once so completely and uniquely filled by that presence. Only when grief extends beyond a healthy length of time, eroding daily life for a prolonged period, should something be done to help the griever.

The Maya Death Ritual Family members make an altar to their loved one containing a photo of the deceased, flowers, white candles, fruits, and sometimes food from each meal. They invite

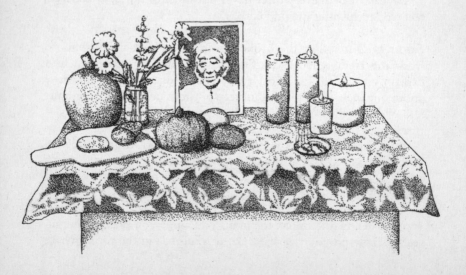

friends and neighbors to spend the entire first night together singing hymns and praying for the departed. This is called the *Belario.*

Usually the deceased is buried by a priest or minister the following day. It is tradition to burn copal incense during the religious rites until the final load of dirt is shoveled over the coffin. Then at sunset the family invites the community to come by to visit in order to pray and sing again for nine consecutive days. Finally, on the ninth evening, a larger group gathers for more prayers, incense, hymns, and a meal that is usually prepared by the neighbors.

On the first anniversary of the passing, family and friends again come together at the deceased's home for another prayer vigil that may last all night. Some families leave the altar with the photo in a prominent place for years. It is considered an honor to tend the altar, change the fruits, freshen the flowers, and attend to the candles.

Remembering the Dead November 1, All Souls' Day, or El Dia de Los Todos Santos, is the day for remembering the dead. All Souls' Day was originally a Celtic tradition that came with Catholicism, and it may well be a combination of modern and ancient customs of the New and the Old Worlds. Nevertheless, it is a lovely tradition and well worth knowing about.

The oldest person in the family recalls all the family members who have passed into the spirit world. Then the women of the family bake a small loaf of bread for each person remembered. The initials of that person are inscribed in strips of dough on the top. During a procession at sunset the breads are carried to the gravesite in a basket. Family members proceed through the streets in large groups, singing hymns, carrying the baskets and lit white candles. It is a beautiful sight to behold and establishes a sense of honor and wonder for the afterlife of the deceased.

At the gravesite the family places each loaf of bread on a piece of cloth or lace and burns white candles while waiting for the blessing of the priest. He comes by with holy water and prayers for each of the graves. The adults pray and burn copal while the children play with each other.

The Maya believe that the dead love to be remembered on this day and that they return from the afterlife to absorb the spiritual

Magic

Most people who talk about magic have no idea what they are talking about. What really is magic? Good magic is good prayer and intent. Bad magic is bad prayer and intent. It is as simple as that.

Prayer and intent are both ch'ulel, or energy, and many studies have shown that energy has an impact on humans, plants, animals, all of life. Whether or not we know it, prayers and intents of all kinds are zooming around us every day. We're used to thinking that someone's mood affects us. Well, prayer and intent are no different. Continued negative thoughts toward one person is a kind of prayer. Even our own depressed thoughts about ourselves are prayers. Conversely, upbeat, hopeful thoughts are prayers for the good.

Through his treatments Don Elijio practiced "good magic" with the intention of giving aid, succor, and assistance to those afflicted with spiritual and physical diseases.

Maldad is evil magic. In Spanish the word *maldad* means evil. Maldad is believed to be intentional evil enchantment, whereas envy and even the evil eye are not often deliberate.

Maldad occurs when one person, feeling angry and jealous of another, hires a practitioner of evil magic to cast an evil spell on that individual. Don Elijio's father, Nicanor, was such a black magician. These cases usually involve unresolved conflict between families or individuals. The aim of the maldad spell is "to get even" with the victim by ensuring his or her failure in life. Maldad magic can also lead to soul possession. The Maya believe that a maldad spell can lead to death if left untreated. Untreated, the web of hatred and evil spreads, and the practitioner becomes more effective and powerful.

The diagnosis and treatment of maldad can be done only by a h'men: it requires the ability to communicate with the spirit world. Through dreams or the sastun, a h'men can confirm the diagnosis of maldad and then use his or her power to lift the evil curse or enchantment.

When Don Elijio introduced me to the concept of maldad, it wasn't easy for me to accept responsibility for dealing with this kind of spiritual illness. I was terrified the first time he had me work with a woman he called "possessed" and asked me to help him perform what amounted to an exorcism on her. I was nearly as horrified when he dragged me along with him to cleanse a house and left me alone with the evil spirits he said were responsible for strange events that had occurred in that household. But over the years I have come to understand how helpful this kind of spiritual intercession can be.

offering of love and remembrance that is in the bread. This is not a time of sadness but of jubilation. It is also the time to request assistance from the ancestors with rain, harvest, healing, family disputes, and other problems.

This kind of community life and ancestral remembrance is sorely lacking in our society, but still we can learn from the Maya and use some of their wisdom in our own grieving process.

Spiritual Illnesses That Require a H'men: Lost Souls of a Deceased Person, Ghosts, Unemployed Spirits, and Spirit Possession

A "lost soul" is a dead person who has not made the complete transition from the physical plane on earth to the realm of the dead in the spirit world. Instead, the person wanders in an intermediary plane the Maya call *Xibalba,* or "the place of awe." Lost souls are usually people who died violently and suddenly and did not have time to prepare for death, to make a confession, to right wrongs, or to have the benefit of prayer as they died.

These unfortunate souls wander in a state of confusion and fright. Some respond to the call of practitioners of evil magic and out of their pain and need become vehicles for evildoing.

"Ghosts" are chronically lost souls who have been wandering in a confused state for years. Because of their great need for companionship and communication, they often inhabit their last place of residence in life.

According to the Maya, lost souls and ghosts are imprisoned in the underworld in the World Tree, where they are neither completely dead nor alive. Like some lost souls, ghosts can also become so desperate that they allow themselves to be used by hechiseros for evil purposes. In extreme cases evil spirits—ghosts or lost souls—can possess living individuals.

A Maya h'men can perform a ritual that helps lost souls and ghosts find their way. The h'men also performs exorcisms.

Self-Help Ritual for the Suddenly Departed   Maya traditional healers say we must always send prayers and spiritual offerings to the dead, especially those who died suddenly. The prayers, they say, soothe the lost souls, protect them from bad company, and call upon angels to guide them gently home to peace.

This is something that you can do yourself. Set up an altar on a tabletop, shelf, or convenient location in the house. You may prefer to have it in a private place to avoid curious questions from visitors. Place a photo of the deceased on the altar along with any religious symbols, statues, or objects appropriate to the faith of the departed. A flower offering is always appropriate, especially white roses or marigolds, but any flowers that you bring to the altar with love are fine.

The flower vase and the altar should be kept clean and fresh at all times. Plan a time when you can sit or kneel before the altar and pray in the manner that is appropriate to you. Catholic Maya say the rosary in front of the altar. Burning incense of copal, sage, cedar, or rosemary purifies and cleanses the atmosphere surrounding the deceased and, according to the Maya, leaves them feeling as if they have been "bathed" in a warm bath. Repeat this every day for nine days. One easy way to count the sessions is to place nine stones in a bowl and to move them one at a time into another bowl until you have completed the nine offerings.

The Maya Healing Garden

With very little garden space you can create your own Maya healing garden from which you can harvest nature's healing bounty for both physical and spiritual ailments. Think of it as your own medicinal plant reserve. Such a garden is for more than personal enjoyment—it contributes to the planet. Natural habitats for medicinal plants are vanishing as more land is developed.

These blessed plants will add beauty to your environment and provide you and your family, friends, and clients with powerful tools for healing common ailments. Using the instructions in this

Creating a Backyard Reserve

Even if you don't want to start a garden, set aside a small patch of your backyard for plants to grow wild. Doing so provides a home for plants that are indigenous to your part of the world and encourages biodiversity. Doing nothing does so much.

book, you can make the plants into herbal teas, soothing herbal baths, salves, cough syrups, and incense.

Starting Your Healing Garden

First decide where your garden will be. Choose a sunny location with average soil. None of these healing plants are fussy, but they need at least eight hours of sun a day, average soil, and consistent watering. Add a good dose of love, and you have a winning combination.

Clear away the weeds, turn the soil, and work some fertilizer or compost into the earth. Do this in early spring or late fall.

Here is a list of easy-to-grow, cooperative plants that can be started from seeds or from pots purchased in nurseries:

Container Garden

If you don't have a backyard, you can make a healing garden in pots on a terrace or windowsill. If you are making a container garden, purchase pots that are about ten inches across and a few bags of potting soil. Fill the containers first with one inch of sand for drainage, then fill with potting soil to one inch below the top of the container.

Rue: from nursery starter
Basil: from nursery starter or seed package
Marigold: from nursery starter or seed package
Rosemary: from nursery starter
Thyme: from nursery starter
Sage: from nursery starter or seed package
Red and white roses: from nursery starter
Amaranth: from seed package (see Resources appendix)
Hibiscus: from nursery starter

Start with one or two of each plant. Rue is usually available in only one variety. Basil has numerous species you can experiment with later, but for now stick with sweet basil. Marigold can be either the dwarf or the tall variety depending on your garden space. The dwarf is nice for containers or borders in front of the other plants, and the tall is better for the inside of the garden. Rosemary, thyme, and sage are usually found in only one domestic variety.

The roses come in bags and should be placed in their own little space along a fence or next to a house wall with plenty of sunlight. Many rose bushes do just fine in containers. Hibiscus also can do well in a large container. Bring it inside near a sunny window during the winter.

You can make each plant its own little bed, which you can separate if you like with stones or small plastic fences. Or you can plant them all in little groups at random.

Roses, hibiscus, and amaranth can grow to about three feet in height. The dwarf marigolds when mature will be six to twelve inches. The rest will grow to about two feet.

Start your seeds indoors in February. This is a good time to lay out a small plan for your garden. It doesn't need to be elaborate and can be just a vision in your head of what you would like your garden to look like. Plants love attention, so it would be nice if you placed your garden where it's easy to show them off and share their beauty.

Planting

When all danger of frost is past, it's time to transplant the seedlings and starter plants. Transplanting is best done on cloudy days or after direct sun is off the garden space in the late afternoon.

Gently—very gently—loosen the soil around the plants and remove them with as much dirt intact as possible from their pots. Prepare a hole in the soil for each plant. Gently place the plant in the hole so that the soil is halfway between the roots and the first leaves. Make sure the roots are covered and the plant is anchored firmly. Tap down the soil around the stem. When all the plants have been transplanted, water them generously with a sprinkler or watering can.

Cultivating

After that first day water the plants in the early morning and evening for a week, then twice weekly after that. Keep your plants free of weeds so that they have space to grow.

Sit with them once in a while—just be there with them. Either out loud or to yourself, tell them that you will be asking them for their help with physical and spiritual ailments. Give them a vote of thanks and appreciation for their healing wonders and promise to take good care of them. Be sure to admire their beauty.

Harvesting

If your plants are thriving, you can begin to harvest them in about thirty days by pinching off leaves and flower heads. Before picking, stop for a moment to recognize them as you would any friend. Explain that you are about to remove some of their leaves and flowers to use as a bath, a tea, or some other remedy. Explain your need and why you are making this remedy and for whom. Give thanks to the plant and state your faith that it will help you achieve what you desire.

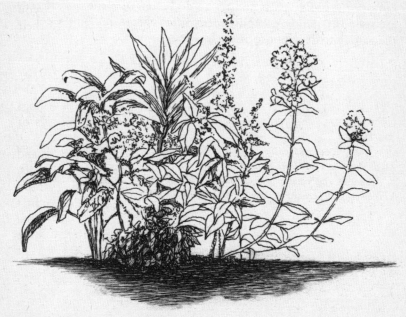

Throughout the summer you can continue to pinch off branches, leaves, and flowers as long as you don't overdo it and put the plant's survival in jeopardy. How much is too much? During midsummer never take any more than one-third of any plant. If there's more than you can use, dry cuttings for the winter months.

Drying Plants

Place the cuttings on old brown paper bags from the grocery store in front of a window where there is plenty of light and circulating air. Another method is to separate them into bunches that you tie up with a string. Hang them from your kitchen beams or ceiling or in a dry basement. Some people place the plants on a cookie tray and bake them in the oven at 100 degrees Fahrenheit for an hour. The plants will come out crisp and dry.

Storing

Store dried plants in paper bags or glass jars in a dry place. Whatever you do, don't let the plants mold. If they begin to mold, remove the moldy parts and try to do better with the rest. If they are seriously moldy, compost them or lay them back on the soil in the garden to decompose on their own.

NOTES

1. Larry Dossey, *Healing Words: The Power of Prayer and the Practice of Medicine* (San Francisco: HarperSanFrancisco, 1993).

2. Sandra Ingerman, *Soul Retrieval: Mending the Fragmented Self* (San Francisco: HarperSanFrancisco, 1991), p. 19.

PART V

Maya Daily Wisdom: Nine Pointers for Healthy Living

Maya villagers generally live a simple lifestyle. They eat what they grow, work hard, and have a community-based life. Before heading to the village health care clinic, they are likely to try a natural home remedy. Since their households are intergenerational, most of them include an elder who can suggest herbal remedies or administer a massage or herbal bath.

It would be nice if we could replicate this lifestyle, but of course we can't! Here are nine pointers that reflect Maya preventive wisdom and will help you live a long, healthy, and useful life. These pointers are not impossible to live by, even in our modern, harried world.

1. Diet

Don't overeat. Stop eating before you feel full. In a few minutes the food in your stomach will expand and you will feel satiated.

Chew your food well. There are no teeth in the stomach. You will get the full nutritional value of your meals only if you chew slowly.

A simple dietary plan to follow is

- 75 percent fruits and vegetables
- 10 percent protein from meat, dairy, beans, or seeds and nuts
- 10 percent whole grains from brown rice, quinoa, millet, or wheat
- 5 percent fat and oil

Whenever possible, eat organically grown foods.

Eliminate as much sugar, dessert, and caffeine as possible from your diet. Try to eat nothing between meals except fruit or nuts, and then only if you are truly hungry.

Don't eat late at night, and allow at least four to six hours
   between meals.
Never miss an opportunity to miss a meal.
Have no more than two alcoholic drinks a day.

2. Water

Drink plenty of plain water. Our bodies need at least eight glasses
daily, and more if we are suffering from any kind of health problem. Drink water at room temperature, not cold.

3. Exercise

Exercise is essential. Love your exercise program so that you will
stick with it. Walking, dancing, swimming, yoga, and lifting weights
are all good. For busy or lazy people, get a stretching video and do it
daily—just thirty minutes a day will change your life. Guaranteed.

4. Natural Remedies

Learn what natural remedies fit your prevention needs. Subscribe
to an herbal magazine and learn about natural therapies to use at
home before you call the doctor.

5. Massage

Get a full-body massage as often as you can afford it. Massage
reduces stress, enhances the immune system, and aids circulation.

6. Feelings

Let out your emotions with a friend. Don't let feelings fester.
Talking helps you to understand yourself better and reduces negative energy.

7. Giving

Share your time and talents with your community. Join up. Volunteer. Giving is rewarding and helps us to focus on someone else's need instead of obsessing about our own. When we reach out to others, somehow our own needs are fulfilled.

8. Breathe!!

It's amazing how rarely we take advantage of the simplest health enhancer we have—oxygen. Every cell in the body requires it, every breath is fuel. Learn deep breathing techniques from a book. Just five minutes a day will strengthen every fiber of your being. This also means: *don't smoke!*

9. Play

Get plenty of rest, figure out what fun means to you, and then have as much of it as possible.

Rosita's Acknowledgments

There is a difference between wisdom and knowledge. I could never give enough credit to those traditional healers who shared their wisdom with me over the past thirty years of living in Central America. It is to them that I owe the bank of accumulated knowledge that they so generously shared with me in the interest of helping people they will never meet. They were potters, saddle makers, seamstresses, herbalists, massage therapists, shamans, midwives, and snake doctors. We have had mutually rewarding relationships over the years.

To the members of the Traditional Healers Foundation:

Don Elijio Panti, Maya h'men, who more than any other traditional healer took me under his wing as apprentice, protégé, and friend. He passed away in 1996 at age 103 after a wonderful life marked by service and genius. On the day he passed the heavens were enriched and the earth was impoverished.

Hortence Robinson, herbal midwife and shaman of Belize, who shared her friendship and her knowledge. Many of the herbal remedies in this book came from her over a ten-year period. Although at times I felt it was like trying to catch feathers in the wind, I did manage to record some of her intuitive genius and experience, gleaned from many generations of healers in her family.

Beatrice Waight, village healer of Belize, who has been generous in her teachings and a good friend over the years. Mother of nine children, Beatrice was trained by her father and grandmothers, who came from Mexico during the Caste Wars, in the old traditions of Yucateca Maya. She is a strong, beautiful woman.

Polo Romero, snake doctor and bushmaster of Belize, who has given me care and guidance while working in the bush for many years collecting plants, sharing knowledge, and rescuing and transplanting medicinal plant species at Terra Nova Forest Reserve.

Thanks also to the traditional healers Juana and Antonio Cuc, who have cared for many generations using plant remedies; Juana Shish, a primary health care specialist in Succotz Village; Barbara Fernandez of Belize City, who has an herb shop in the Belize City market that is well known and respected throughout the country and who wrote *Medicine Woman: The Herbal Tradition of Belize;* Thomas Green of Cayo District, who learned his trade in the chicle, rubber, and mahogany camps and is an accomplished canoe craftsman as well; Percival Reynolds, now deceased, who liked to be known as a "scientific herbalist"; Winston Harris of Cristo Rey Village in Cayo, known as a master of jungle survival as well as a snakebite healer; Andrew Ramcharon, famous snake doctor of Calcutta in Corozal District, who was trained by his father and grandfather from Calcutta, India; and Artita Guerra, potter and traditional healer of Durazno, Guerrero, in southern Mexico.

I could only wish that every writer had such a patient and amenable muse as Nadine Epstein, my friend and faithful cowriter. I'm a better writer and person for having known her. Thanks too to Noah Phillips for showing patience while his mom spent hours with me at the computer.

To my husband, Greg Shropshire, for the innumerable ways he has loved and supported me over the past twenty years.

To my children—James Arvigo, James Cimarolli, and Crystal Arvigo—for they represent the lessons of the past, the hope of the future, and the reason for the present. Special thanks go to Crystal Arvigo for managing affairs at Ix Chel Farm, making it possible for me to be away from Belize for long periods of time while writing this book.

To my aunt Emma Eshoo Ashford for being a wild woman.

To Michael J. Balick, director of the Institute of Economic Botany and associate director of the New York Botanical Garden, for teaching us to be good ethnobotanists and field researchers. To him I owe a great debt. He introduced me to the world of science and plants, which made my love for herbology and healing grow like the forest around us. To his assistant, Liz Pecchia, for her patience and help over the years, and to Willa Capraro for most valuable assistance with so many aspects of the Belize Ethnobotany Project (BEP). United States Aid to International Development (USAID) funded the nine years of the BEP to collect medicinal plants in Belize for cancer and AIDS research in Washington, during which time some of the information in this book was gathered. Thanks also for the support received from the U.S. Cancer Institute and Dr. Gordon Cragg, the Rockefeller Foundation, the Metropolitan Life Insurance Foundation, the Overbrook Foundation, the Edward John Noble Foundation, the Philecology Trust, the Rex Foundation, the John D. and Catherine T. MacArthur Foundation, and the Nathan Cummings Foundation.

To Patty and Matt Long, along with the Gildea Foundation, for their generous support of our Children's Bush Medicine Camp—may the Maya spirits reward them. Thanks also to Emery, Patrick, and Dorothy Long, intrepid campers.

To Hugh O'Brien, director of Central Farm in Belize, former principal of the Belize College of Agriculture, and director of the Medicinal Plants Committee in Belize, for his support and confidence in our work during even the roughest times.

To Raphael Manzanero, Earl Green, Richard Belisle, Oscar Rosado, Daniel Silva, Francisco Salazar, John Link, John Pinelo, Carol August, Melanie Santiago, Dennis Jones and The Belize Enterprise for Sustainable Technology, Bridget Cullerton, and Ainslie Leslie.

To my longtime friend, sister, and collaborator, Colletta Aberdale, for her brilliance, devotion, and loyalty over the years.

To Mick, Lucy, Piers, Bryony, and Ann Fleming for being good pals and good neighbors over the decades. Those afternoon teas and overnight respites kept me going.

To the staff at Ix Chel Tropical Research Foundation: Tara Blanco Gamero, Rigoberto Gamero, Ruth Guittierez Coh, Ruth Pech, Pablo Cocom, Rolando Cocom, Vivian Tzib, Belarmino Mai, Auxiliadora, and Rigoberto Pech.

To the Forestry Department and Conservation Division, Belize Ministry of Natural Resources, for permits to collect plants and for their support, without which little would have been possible.

To my heroes and heroines: Ethel Arvigo, Sharon Matola, Patch Adams, Katie Valk, Rosemary Gladstar, Gail Ulrich, Brigitte Mars, Marion Rose, Feather Jones, Diana DeLuca, Christa Obuchowski, Jim Duke, Mark Blumenthal, Katy Moran, Steve King, Norman Farnsworth, Al Kapuler, Sue Clemens, Janice Alcorn, Trish Flaster, Seven Song, Pam Montgomery, Varro Tyler, Mindi Green, Michael Tierra, Susun Weed, Janice Longboat, Timothy Plowman, and Ann Bradburn.

To Bob and Nettie Jones of Eva's Restaurant in San Ignacio, Cayo, for a million favors and countless laughs.

To numerous individuals at the New York Botanical Garden: Daniel Atha, Noah Goldstein, Hans Beck, Brian Boom, Mee Young Choi, Willa Capraro, Douglas Daly, Gregory Long, and Michael Nee; and to the staff of the herbarium and library, as well as the botanists of the Institute of Systematic Botany and their fellow systematists around the world who have identified many of the plants mentioned in this book.

To Frontier Herbs of Norway, Iowa, and Nick Frost of Santa Fe, New Mexico, and the Bioneers Institute for their support of Traditional Healers Foundation projects.

Finally, but certainly not least, to the trees and plants of Belize— collectively you are my mentors, healers, counselors, companions, and raison d'être. I trust that our efforts on your behalf somewhat reflect your efforts on our behalf. I pray that you will have a real future of protection and respect in Belize, in Central America, and throughout the world.

Thanks to the Nine Maya Spirits, especially Ix Chel, for their dream visions and attention to me over the years.

Ix Chel Farm, Belize

Nadine's
Acknowledgments

To Rosita Arvigo, for being a wonderful friend, houseguest, cowriter, coadventurer, and colearner. As always, working with her and the Maya spirits has been a joy and an honor.

To Bridget Gazo, librarian of pre-Columbian studies at Harvard University's Dumbarton Oaks Library in Washington, D.C., for letting us make use of this amazing resource. The books we found on the Dumbarton Oaks shelves enriched this book and each of us. To Sandra Parker-Provenzano and Toni Stephens for their cheerful assistance.

To Charles Eisendrath of the Michigan Journalism Fellows Program and Max Heirich of the University of Michigan for making it possible for me to study mind-body medicine in 1989–90. Assignments from *Smithsonian* and *Ms.* magazines, and the *Whole Earth Review* led me to Belize.

Wise advice was given by all our readers: the archaeologist Anabel Ford, the shaman-apprentice Caroline Kenner, the writer Debra Bruno, the ethnobotanist Michael Balick, the therapist Deborah Fox, the acupuncturist Margaret Beatty, the internist and acupuncturist Ali Safayan, the natural healer and EMT Gregory Shropshire, and the naprapath Sheila Leidy. Anthropologist James Boster provided further insight into Maya healing.

The staffs of Ix Chel Farm and the Bush Medicine Camp went out of their way to make us comfortable during our stay in Belize. Patty Long made bush medicine camp possible—and included Noah. Special thanks to Dorothy Long for being such a good pal for Noah: he had a great time sleeping under the table too. To Crystal Arvigo, she is wise beyond her years.

To our agent, Al Zuckerman, and his assistant, Faye Greenfield, and editors Karen Levine, Doug Abrams, and especially Renee Sedliar for help making this book a reality.

To many dear friends: Linda Feldmann, Rebecca and Evan Roe, Eileen Dzik, Jack Edelstein, Lisa Newman, Jan Genzer, Lonni Moffet, David McCandlish, Georgia Moffet-McCandlish, Monica Bussolati, E. R. Shipp, Tracey Steiner, Laurent Amzallag, Arlene Dookwah, Joe Dempsey, Sharon Gillooly, Evan and Claire Dempsey, Natasha Nenadovic and Marcus, Gloria, and Mike Levitas, Deborah Fox, Bob and Claudia Schwebel, Teresa Leal, Lucinda and Sydney LaRee, and the Cavalieri-Grosse family. Thank you.

To James Bronson: He found innumerable kind ways to help.

To Donald and Jeanne Epstein, Mildred Epstein, Marcy Epstein, Michael Epstein, and my parents—Ruth and Seymour—for their support and encouragement.

To John O'Leary: He rescued lost computer files, hand-fed hundreds of pages of paper into the printer, kept me informed about the news, and made me laugh.

To Noah Phillips: He is a joy to all, and was patient with a mom who monopolized the computer so that he couldn't play *Carmen Sandiego* as much as he would have liked.

Washington, D.C.

Latin Names of Plants

Allspice: *Pimenta dioica*
Aloe: *Aloe vera*
Amanth: *Amaranthus retroflexus*
Avocado: *Persea americana*
Balsam: *Myroxylon balsaminum*
Banana: *Musa acuminata*
Basil: *Ocimum basilicum*
Bitter gourd: *Momordica charantia*
Bullhorn acacia: *Acacia cornigera*
Burdock: *Arctium lappa*
Ceiba: *Ceiba pentandra*
Chamomile: *Matricaria recutita* or *Anthemis nobilis*
Chayote: *Sechium edule*
Chicle or sapodilla tree: *Achras zapota*
China root: *Smilax lanceolata*
Cinnamon: *Cinnamomum*
Clove: *Eugenia caryophyllata*
Copal: *Protium copal*
Corn silk: *Zea mays*
Damiana: *Turnera aphrodisiaca*
Dandelion: *Taraxacum officinalis*

Elderberry: *Sambucus nigra*
Epazote (Mexican wormseed): *Chenopodium ambrosioides*
Garlic: *Allium sativum*
Ginger: *Zingiber officinale*
Guaco: *Aristolochia odoratissima*
Guinweo: *Agonandra*
Gumbo-limbo: *Bursera simaruba*
Hibiscus: *Hibiscus rosa-sinensis*
Hollyhock: *Althaea rosea*
Horsetail: *Equisetum arvense*
Jackass bitters: *Neurolaena lobata*
Jewelweed: *Impatiens capensis*
Kava kava: *Piper methysticum*
Lemongrass: *Cymbopogon citratus*
Life everlasting: *Kalanchoe pinnata*
Man vine: *Agonandra racemosa*
Marigold: *Tagetes erecta* and related species
Melissa: *Melissa officinalis*
Mexican wild yam: *Dioscorea*
Mexican wormseed (epazote): *Chenopodium ambrosioides*

Motherwort: *Leonurus cardiaca*
Nopal: *Opuntia cochenillifera*
Onion: *Allium cepa*
Orange: *Citrus reticulata*
Oregano: *Lippia graveolens*
Papaya: *Carica papaya*
Parsley: *Petroselinum crispum*
Passionflower: *Passiflora incarnata*
Peppermint: *Mentha piperita*
Plantain (the banana): *Musa paradisiaca*
Plantain (the herb): *Plantago*
Potato: *Solanum tuberosum*
Pumpkin: *Cucurbita pepo*
Purslane: *Portulaca oleracea*
Radish: *Raphanus sativus*
Red clover: *Trifolium pratense*
Rose, red: *Rosa chinensis*
Rosemary: *Rosmarinus officinalis*
Rosy periwinkle: *Catharanthus roseus*
Rue: *Ruta graveolens*
Sage: *Salvia officinalis*
Saint-John's-wort: *Hypericum perforatum*
Saw palmetto: *Serenoa repens*
Sensitive plant: *Mimosa pudica*
Sesame: *Sesamum indicum*
Skunk root: *Chiococca alba*
Squaw vine: *Mitchella repens*
Stinging nettle: *Urtica dioica*
Strong back: *Desmodium adscendens*
Thyme: *Thymus vulgaris*
Vervain: *Stachytarpheta cayennensis*
Yarrow: *Achillea millefolium*
Yellow dock: *Rumex crispus*

Resources

TO ORDER HERBS AND REMEDIES FROM BELIZE

Rainforest Remedies

    Ix Chel Farm
    San Ignacio, Cayo, Belize
    ixchel@btl.net
    www.ixchelherbs
    www.rainforestremedies.com
    http://members.aol.com/RainfstRem

[handwritten annotations: IX, Sacred Feminine, Wise Women, Goddess, Chel, Rainbow]

Agape Herbs

    PO Box 1608
    Belize City, Belize
    Central America

Aunt Barbara Fernandez

    Back to Eden Herb Stall
    Old Market
    Belize City, Belize
    Central America

TO ORDER TINCTURES

For wholesale orders:

Lotus Light Enterprises, Inc.

PO Box l008
Silver Lake, WI 52170
414–889–8501
414–889–8591 (fax)
800–548–3824 (orders)

For retail orders:

Internatural

33719 116th St.
Twin Lakes, WI 53181
414–889–8581
800–643–4221 (orders)
www.internatural.com

The tinctures available include Flex Free, Belly Be Good, Nerve Support, Back Support, Cold Season, Strong Resistance, Clearing Support, Female Tonic, and Male Tonic. Charcoal to burn incense is also available.

TO ORDER DRIED HERBS

For both retail and wholesale orders:

Colletta Aberdale

43 Beacon St.
Northampton, MA 100l6
colletta@javanet.com

Dried herbs available are jackass bitters, gumbo-limbo, skunk root, man vine root, wild yam, China root, and strong back. Also available are Miss Hortence's Special Female Formula, copal incense, Maya Moon Oil, insect repellent, Jungle Salve, Traveler's Tonic, and Kidney Tonic.

TO ORDER PSORIASIS AND ECZEMA CREAM

Dan Wagner

Nutrifarmacy
2506 Wildwood Rd.
Wildwood, PA 15091
1–877–289–7478
dtwmedi@aol.com
www.nutrifarmacy.com

FOR INFORMATION ABOUT MAYA
ABDOMINAL MASSAGE WORKSHOPS

Colletta Aberdale

43 Beacon St.
Northampton, MA 10016
colletta@javanet.com

Colletta Aberdale can also help you locate practitioners of Maya abdominal massage in your area.

FOR INFORMATION ABOUT MAYA HEALTH
AND HEALING SEMINARS

Ix Chel Tropical Research Foundation and
Traditional Healers Foundation

Ix Chel Farm
San Ignacio, Cayo
Belize
011–501–923–870
ixchel@btl.net

Ix Chel Farm can also give you information about Traditional Healers Foundation of Belize, the *Tree of Life* newsletter, the Terra Nova Forest Reserve and Tree Planting Camp Program, and the Bush Medicine Camp for Children. Donations are also accepted at this address.

FOR MORE INFORMATION ABOUT HERBS AND HERBAL PRODUCTS

American Botanical Council

PO Box 201660
Austin, TX 78720
512–331–1924

HerbalGram magazine

PO Box 144345
Austin, TX 78714–4335
512–926–4900
800–373–7105
www.herbalgram.org

Herb Research Foundation

1007 Pearl St., Suite 200
Boulder, CO 80302
303–449–2265
www.herbs.org

TO LOCATE A DOCTOR OF NAPRAPATHY IN YOUR AREA

Chicago National College of Naprapathy

3330 N. Milwaukee Ave.
Chicago, IL 60633
312–282–2686

TO PURCHASE UNUSUAL SEEDS

Seeds of Change

2385 SE Thompson St.
Corvalis, OR 97333–1919

HERBS AVAILABLE AT SPANISH STORES

Epazote
Red roses *(rosas)*
Rue *(ruda)*
Rosemary *(romero)*
Nopal
Vervain *(verbena)*
Chayote
Lemongrass *(zacate limon)*

HERBAL PRODUCTS AVAILABLE FROM
RAINFOREST REMEDIES COMPANY

All plants used in the extracts are wild-crafted from tropical rain-forest areas cited for development. All sales help to support Ix Chel Tropical Research Foundation in Belize, the Traditional Healers Foundation, the Terra Nova Forest Reserve, educational programs in Belize schools and the Bush Medicine Camp for Children.

Belly Be Good For gastritis, constipation, and chronic gas pains. Ingredients: man vine, guinweo, guaco, cane alcohol, water.

Blood Tonic For anemia, toxic blood, rheumatism, and arthritis. Sold as "Flex Free" in the U.S. market. Ingredients: China root, wild yam.

Detox Formula To tone organs and detoxify the blood. Sold as "Clearing Support" in the U.S. market. Ingredients: chicoloro, Billy Webb, jackass bitters, guaco, cane alcohol, water.

Female Tonic For painful periods, PMS, uterine conditions, and menopause. Ingredients: China root, copalchi, man vine, Billy Webb, skunk root, ginger, wild yam, cane alcohol, water.

Flu-Away To be taken at first signs of cold or flu. Sold as "Cold Season" in the U.S. market. Ingredients: jackass bitters, garlic, cayenne, cane alcohol, water.

Immune Boost For colds, flu, infections, and exposure to infectious diseases. Sold as "Strong Resistance" in the U.S. market. Ingredients: Billy Webb, jackass bitters, John Charles, cane alcohol, water.

Insect Repellent Ingredients: aloe vera, bitter herbs, essential oils, lecithin.

Jungle Salve For insect bites, itching, poison ivy, poison wood, skin irritations, and rashes. Ingredients: jackass bitters, gumbo-limbo, chicoloro, pure vegetable oil, and beeswax.

Kidney Tonic For all urinary complaints, water retention, and liver ailments. Ingredients: balsam bark, corn silk, wild yam, cane alcohol, water.

Male Tonic For male virility, kidney, and bladder complaints. Ingredients: balsam bark, corn silk, man vine root, cane alcohol, water.

Maya Moon Oil A special blend with essential oils and nine sacred Maya plants collected during the full-moon phase with prayers. An all-purpose oil for massage, skin, hair, and so on.

Nerve Tonic For stress, anxiety, and insomnia. Sold as "Nerve Support" in the U.S. market. Ingredients: man vine, cane alcohol, water.

Pressure For moderately high blood pressure, poor circulation, and high cholesterol. Ingredients: juarumo, chayote, garlic, cane alcohol, water.

Strong Back For backache, muscle spasms, and athletic strain, and to halt the onset of asthma. Sold as "Back Support" in the U.S. market. Ingredients: strong back, wild yam, man vine, cane alcohol, water.

Sunburn Ointment For fresh sunburn or kitchen burns. Ingredients: aloe vera, bitter herbs, vegetable shortening, beeswax.

Sweet Blood For diabetes, dry cough, and low appetite. Ingredients: Billy Webb bark, cane alcohol, water.

Traveler's Tonic For amoebas, diarrhea, parasites, and salmonella. Ingredients: jackass bitters, guava leaf, cane alcohol, water.

Bibliography

Aman. 1979. *Medical Secrets of Your Food.* Mysore, India: Wesley Press.

Arvigo, Rosita. 1998. "Maya Uterine and Abdominal Massage." Unpublished manuscript. San Ignacio, Belize.

Arvigo, Rosita, and Michael J. Balick. 1994. *Rainforest Remedies: One Hundred Healing Herbs of Belize.* Twin Lakes, WI: Lotus Press.

Arvigo, Rosita, and Nadine Epstein. 1994. *Sastun: My Apprenticeship with a Maya Healer.* San Francisco: HarperSanFrancisco.

Ayensu, E. S. 1981. *Medicinal Plants of the West Indies.* Algonac, MI: Reference Publications.

Badianus Manuscript: An Aztec Herbal of 1552. 1940. Baltimore: Johns Hopkins University Press.

Berlin, Brent, and Elois Berlin. 1996. *Medical Ethnobotany of the Highland Maya of Chiapas, Mexico: The Gastrointestinal Disease.* Princeton, NJ: Princeton University Press.

Boster, James. *Kiekchii Maya, Curing Practiasin.* British Honduras: Harvard University, 1973.

Chaiken, Miriam. *Menorahs, Mezuzas, and Other Jewish Symbols.* New York: Clarion Books, 1990.

Colby, Benjamin N., and Lore M. Colby. 1981. *The Daykeeper: The Life and Discourse of an Ixil Diviner.* Cambridge, MA: Harvard University Press.

Dossey, Larry. 1993. *Healing Words: The Power of Prayer and the Practice of Medicine.* San Francisco: HarperSanFrancisco.

———. 1996. *Prayer Is Good Medicine.* San Francisco: HarperSanFrancisco.

Douglas, Bill Gray. 1969. "Illness and Curing in Santiago Atitlan: A Tzutujil Maya Community in the Southwest Highlands of Guatemala." Ph.D. dissertation, Stanford University.

Duke, Jim. 1997. *The Green Pharmacy.* Emmaus, PA: Rodale Press.

Eliade, Mircea. 1967. *From Muhammed to Medicine Men.* New York: Harper & Row.

Fabrega, M., Jr., and Daniel Ben Silver. 1973. *Illness and Shamanistic Curing in Zinzcantan: An Ethnomedical Analysis.* Stanford, CA: Stanford University Press.

Foster, George W. 1994. *Hippocrates' Latin American Legacy: Humoral Medicine in the New World.* Berkeley, Calif.: Gordon and Breach Science Publishers.

Freidel, David, Linda Schele, and Joy Parker. 1993. *Maya Cosmos: Three Thousand Years on the Shaman's Path.* New York: William Morrow.

Gilbert, A., and M. Cotterell. 1995. *The Mayan Prophecies.* Rockport, MA: Element Books.

Girard, R. 1979. *Esotericism of the Popol Vuh.* Pasadena, CA: Theosophical University Press.

Harner, Michael. 1980. *The Way of the Shaman.* San Francisco: Harper & Row.

Ingerman, Sandra. 1991. *Soul Retrieval: Mending the Fragmented Self.* San Francisco: HarperSanFrancisco.

Jackson, M., and T. Teague. 1982. *The Handbook of Alternatives to Chemical Medicine.* Oakland, CA: Teague & Jackson.

Kay, M. A. 1996. *Healing with Plants in the American and Mexican West.* Tucson: University of Arizona Press.

Kunz, J., and A. Finkel. 1987. *The American Medical Association Family Medical Guide.* Rev. ed. New York: Random House.

Middleton, J. 1967. *Magic, Witchcraft, and Curing.* Austin: University of Texas Press.

Morley, Sylvanus G., and G. W. Brainerd. 1983. *The Ancient Maya.* Stanford, CA: Stanford University Press.

Peredo, M. G. 1992. *Medical Practices in Ancient America.* Mexico: Euroamerican Editions.

Reichel-Dolmatoff, G. 1990. *The Sacred Mountain of Columbian Kogi Indians:* E. J. Brill.

Robineau, L. 1991. *Towards a Caribbean Pharmacopeia:* TRAMIL.

Rogers, S. *The Shamanic Healing Way.* Ramona, CA: Acoma Books.

Shaw, R. J. 1994. *The Ancient Maya.* Stanford, CA: Stanford University Press.

Silver, Daniel Ben. 1966. "Zinacanteco Shamanism." Ph.D. dissertation, Harvard University.

Simons, A., B. Hasselbring, and M. Castleman. 1993. *Before You Call the Doctor.* New York: Fawcett Columbine.

Stevens, J. L. 1969. *Incidents of Travel in Central America, Chiapas, and Yucatan.* Vols. 1 and 2. New York: Dover Publications.

Taylor, L. 1998. *Herbal Secrets of the Rainforest.* Rocklin, CA: Prima Health.

Tedlock, Barbara. *Dreaming: Anthropology and Psychology Interpretations.* Santa Fe, NM: School of American Research Press.

Tedlock, Dennis, trans. 1985. *Popol Vuh: The Definitive Edition of the Mayan Book of the Dawn of Life and the Glories of Gods and Kings.* New York: Touchstone/Simon & Schuster.

Veeris, D. 1999. *Green Remedies and Golden Customers of Our Ancestors.* The Hague, Netherlands: Triangel Publicaties.

Vogel, H. C. A. 1991. *The Nature Doctor: A Manual of Traditional and Complementary Medicine.* New Canaan, CT: Keats Publishing.

Vogel, V. J. 1970. *American Indian Medicine.* Norman: University of Oklahoma Press.

Index

Page numbers of illustrations appear in italics.

Acne, 44
Acupressure: blood circulation, normalizing, 72; ear infections, 120; sore throat, 82
Allspice: berry, for toothache, 86; ointment for foot fungus, 69; poultice for backache, 50; tea, for childbirth, 95; tea, for colic, 116
Aloe vera: burns, 55; constipation, 61–62; cuts and scrapes, 62; insect stings, bites, 75; mouthwash, 70; sulfur powder and, for ringworm, 81; swelling, 86
Amaranth, 46, 48; Asian-Style, 47; cuts and scrapes, 63; Fresh, Broth and Honey, 47; greens and seeds, 105; history of, 105; Rosita's Italian-Style, 47
Amenorrhea, 91–93
Amulets, 38–39, 173–74
Anemia, 45–46
Anger, and liver ailments, 78
Antibiotics, natural, 125–28
Anti-itch salve, 75
Anxiety, teas for, 64
Appetite loss, 146
Applesauce, for diarrhea, 119
Asthma, 48–49, 114–15

Avocado: cream, for wrinkles, 89; osteoporosis, 106

Back ache or pain, 35, 49–50
Bad luck, 174
Baking soda: insect stings, bites, 75; poison ivy, 79
Banana: fresh, for diarrhea, 119; leaf poultice, for burns, 56
Basic principles of Maya medicine, 5–19
Basic tools of Maya healing, 29–39
Basil: bath, for fever, 121; cuts and scrapes, 63; dysmenorrhea, 98; ear infections, 120; fright, 167, *167*; herbal bath for spiritual illness, 160, 170, 179; house cleansing, 177; insect stings, bites, 75; as natural antibiotic for skin infections, 127–28; PMS, 108; powder, 127; ringworm, 81; rinse, 127; -water sweep, 174
Beef lard and honey, as natural antibiotic for skin infections, 128
Belly Be Good, 84
Black beans, for boils, 122
Bladder infections, 51–52
Blood and bloodletting, 16–17, 36
Blood circulation, normalizing, 72
Blood pressure. *See* High blood pressure
Bodywork and massage. *See* Massage
Boils, 122, 123

Breath, 195
Bronchitis and chronic cough, 52–53
Brown sugar and lemon for acne, 44
Bruises, 53–54
Bullhorn tree ants, 118
Burdock, detoxing with, 45
Burns, minor, 54–56

Cabbage: juice, raw, for ulcers, 87; leaf
    poultice, for carpal tunnel, 57–58
Carpal tunnel syndrome, 56–58, 57
Castor oil: child's purge, 122; orange
    juice and, for constipation, 62;
    Plantar warts, 89
Catholic holy water, 175
Catnip tea, for child's sleeplessness, 125
Cayenne: garlic, and jackass bitters
    tincture for colds and flu, 59;
    mouthwash, 70
Cedar incense, 174
Chamomile: flower tea, for colic, 116;
    mouthwash, 70; as natural antibiotic
    for skin infections, 127; relaxing tea,
    74; styes, 84–85; tea, for children's
    sleeplessness, 125
Chanul, 6
Chayote, 75; for high blood pressure, 74
Childbirth, 94–97; bleeding, excessive, 96;
    delivery, 95–96; later pregnancy, 94;
    morning sickness, 94; postdelivery,
    96–97; spotting during pregnancy,
    94–95; tearing, how to avoid, 95
Children and infants: fright in, 164, 165;
    massage, 147–49, 148; physical
    ailments, 114–28; soul loss in, 154
China root (sarsaparilla): impotency,
    114; and wild yam, for gout, 71
Ch'ulel (life energy), 5–7, 16, 155;
    biology of, 156–57; blood and
    bloodletting, 16–17, 36; dreams as
    conduits of, 37; hot and cold and,
    18; incense and, 38; in medicinal
    plants, 31–32; negative, 173–74, 175,
    176, 194; water and, 33, 155–56
Christmas candle (senna plant) for
    fever, 66

Cinnamon: red hibiscus flowers and,
    tea, for bleeding, excessive, after
    childbirth, 96; red hibiscus flowers
    and, tea, for diarrhea, 64; tea, for
    diarrhea, 119
Cleansing a house of envy or bad luck,
    175–77
Colds and flu, 58–61, 117–18. See also
    Bronchitis; Cough syrup
Colic, 115–17
Constipation, 61–62, 115, 146
Copal, 38; incense, 162, 166, 171, 174,
    179
Corn, 13, 14, 14; ceremonies (primicias),
    14–15, 37; prostate enlargement,
    111; recreating of creation through,
    13; starch, for skin rashes, 124
Corn silk: Indian, tea for bladder
    infection, 51; tea, for genito-urinary
    tract (men), 110; tea, for impotency,
    113
Coughs, 117–18; Grannie's Dandelion,
    Syrup, 117; remedy, 117; syrup, all-
    purpose Mayan, 53
Counseling, 34
Cramps: dysmenorrhea, 97–98;
    stomach, 18
Cumin tea, for morning sickness, 94
Cuts and scrapes, 62–63

Dairy products, 91
Dan Wagner's Salve, 80
Dandelion: detoxing with, 45; Grannie's
    Cough Syrup, 117; as natural
    antibiotic for skin infections, 128
Death of a loved one, 182–85; self-help
    ritual for the suddenly departed,
    185–86
Depression (sadness, tristeza), 169–71;
    bath, 103–4; case history from New
    York, 170; menopause-related, 103;
    severe, chronic, treatment for,
    170–71; special ancient treatments,
    169; symptoms, 169
Desert nopal, 18; burns, 56; childbirth,
    95; headache, 73

Diarrhea, 63–64, 118–19
Diet and dietary plan, 193–94
Don Elijio's anti-ciro remedy, 83–84
Dream visions, 37–38

Ear infections, 119–20
Eggplant leaves, and oregano for burns, 54
Egg yolk, raw, for acne, 44
Elderberry tea and peppermint, for colds and flu, 58
Emotions, 194. *See also* Spiritual illness
Endometriosis, 98–99
Endometritis, 99
Envy (*Invidia*), 171–77; amulets, 173–74; cleansing a house of, 175–77; how it works, 172; how we invite envy, 173; special treatments, ancient, 173; symptoms, 172–73; what to do with feelings of, 174
Epazote (Mexican wormseed): colic with constipation, 115; for hangover, 72; for intestinal parasites, 77–78
Estrogen, 99–100
Evil eye, 176
Exercise, 194

Fainting, 65–66
Faith, 156
Female tonic, 103, 108
Fever, 66–67, 121–22
Fibroids, 99–100
Foot rub, 71
Fright (Susto), 163–69; case history, from the Ukraine, 165–66, 168; case history, in utero, 168; guidelines for diagnosis, 163, 165; events that can cause, 164; prayer for, 168–69
Fungus, 67–69

Gallstones, 69–70
Garden. *See* Maya healing garden
Garlic: cayenne, and jackass bitters tincture for colds and flu, 59; ear infections, 120; honey-, 126; for intestinal parasites, 77; as natural antibiotic, 125–26; olive oil-, 126; onion, and honey, for colds and flu, 61; and oregano tea for bronchitis, 52; raw, 126; toenail fungus remedy, 69; warts, 88–89
Gas pains, 84
Gastritis, 146
Ginger: for headache, 73; and lemon, for diarrhea with stomach cramps and vomiting, 118; for stomach cramps, 18; tea for childbirth, 96; tea for colds and flu, 60–61; tea for dysmenorrhea, 98
Gingivitis, 70
Giving, 195
Gout, 70–71
Grannie's Dandelion Cough Syrup, 117
Grief (*pesar*), 177–85; case history from Canada, 178–79; broken hearts, 179–82; death of a loved one, 182–85, *182*; remembering the death, 183, 185; symptoms, 177–78
Guaco vine, for stomach complaints, 83
Guinweo vine, for stomach complaints, 83
Gumbo-limbo tree: as natural antibiotic, 126–27; salve, for poison ivy, 79; and wild yam tea, for psoriasis and eczema, 80

Hangover, 71–72
Headache, 72–74
Healers, types of, 27–29
Heartburn, 146
Herbal baths (hydrotherapy), 33; broken heart, 180–81; colds and flu, 59; skin infections, 123; skin rashes, 124; for spiritual illness, 160–62, 170
Herbal teas, for amenorrhea, 93
Herbs, aromatic: for fainting, 66; for fever, 67
Herbs, detoxifying: acne, 45; gout, 71; infertility, 101

Hibiscus: for bleeding, excessive, after childbirth, 96; cinnamon and, tea, for diarrhea, 64; dysmenorrhea, 97–98; endometritis, 99; headache, 73; newborn bath, 124; and rose lotion, for wrinkles, 89–90, 89; spotting during pregnancy, 94; tonic (Red Zinger tea) for anemia, 46

High blood pressure, 74

Hollyhock flowers, for spotting during pregnancy, 94–95

Honey: beef lard and, as natural antibiotic for skin infections, 128; Fresh Amaranth Broth and, for anemia 47; -garlic, as natural antibiotic, 126; garlic, onion, and, for colds and flu, 61; lemon juice, for colds, flu, 59–60; ulcers, 87

Horsetail tea, for bladder infection, 51–52

Hot and cold, theory of, 18. See also Temperature change, effects of

Humor, 34

Ice pack, for insect stings, bites, 75

Impotency, 112–13

Incense, 38; for broken heart, 181–82; for spiritual illness, 162, 166, 171, 174

Indigestion. See Stomach complaints

Infants. See Children and infants

Infection: foods to avoid, 85; internal, natural antibiotics for, 125–27

Infertility, 100–101

Injuries, 35

Insect bites and stings, 74–75

Insomnia, 75–76

Intestinal parasites, 77–79

Jackass bitters (tres puntas): douche, for vaginitis, 108–9; garlic, cayenne, and, tincture for colds and flu, 59; for intestinal parasites, 77; as natural antibiotic, 126; skin infections, 122–23; tea, for fungus, 69; wound powder, 123

Jewelweed, for poison ivy, 79

Kava kava (piper) for insomnia, 76

Laxatives, 61–62, 66

Lemon: bruises, 54; and ginger, for diarrhea with stomach cramps and vomiting, 118; juice and honey for colds, flu, 59–60; juice, for insect stings, bites, 75; liver ailments, 78

Lemongrass tea, for fever, 66, 121

Life everlasting plant: for asthma, 48–49, 114–15

Liver ailments, 78

Love and broken hearts, 179–82

Magic and maldad (bad magic), 184

Mano, 39

Man vine: impotency, 113; stomach complaints, 83

Marigold: flower tea, for colic, 118; fright (susto), 167, 167; herbal bath, 59; herbal bath for fever, 121; herbal bath for spiritual illness, 160, 179; house cleansing, 177; for insect stings, bites, 75; as natural antibiotic for skin infections, 128; seed tea, for prostate pain, 111

Massage, 34, 131–49, 194; abdominal, 92, 94, 146–47; acne, 44–45; belly rub for colic, 117, 117; carpal tunnel, 57, 57; children's, 147–49, 148; ear infections, 120; five-minute tummy ache massage for infants and children, 149; gout, 71; impotency, 114; prostate, 112, 142–46, 144–45; stomach complaints, 83; uterine, 97, 132–42, 133–35, 138, 139–40

Maya healing garden, 186–90; container garden, 187; creating a backyard reserve, 186; cultivating, 188–89; drying plants, 190; harvesting, 189, 189; plant list, 187; planting, 188; starting, 187–88; storing plants, 190

Maya healing terms, xvi

Mayan death ritual, 182–83, 182

Medicinal plants (xiv), 31–32, 43

Men: abdominal massage for, 146–47; physical ailments, 109–14, see also *specific ailments*; prostate massage, 142–46, *144–45*

Menopause, 102–4; calcium foods for, 102; depression during, 103

Menstruation, 91; amenorrhea, 91–93; dysmenorrhea, 97–98; irregularity, 104

Migraine remedy, Mayan, 73

Miss Hortense's Tea, 115

Morning sickness, 94

Mother's milk and bread, for boils, 123

Motherwort, *101*; endometriosis, 98–99; for insect stings, bites, 75; uterine cleansing, 101

Mouthwash, 70

Nausea, 83, 94

Nettle: root, prostate enlargement, 111–12; stinging, root extract, prostate enlargement, 112

Nightmares, night terrors, 157–58

Numbers, 11, *11*

Okra: for childbirth, 95; dysmenorrhea, 98

Olive oil: dry skin, 65; ear infections, 120; -garlic, as natural antibiotic, 126

Onion: garlic and honey, for colds and flu, 61; juice and honey for bronchitis, 52; liver ailments, 78; milk for bladder infection, 51

Orange: hangover remedy, 71–72; juice and castor oil for constipation, 62; nausea, 83, 94

Oregano: dysmenorrhea, 98; ear infections, 120; and eggplant leaves, for burns, 54; and garlic tea for bronchitis, 52; as natural antibiotic for skin infections, 128; tea bath for bruises, 54

Osteoporosis, 104–6

Papaya: for high blood pressure, 74; seeds, for intestinal parasites, 77; warts, 88

Parasites, 77–79

Parsley for liver ailments, 78

Peppermint: and elderberry tea, for colds and flu, 58, 59; nausea, 83; stomach complaints, 84; toothpaste, for insect stings, bites, 75

Pinchar, 36

Plantain, *87*; ulcers, 87–88

Play, 195

Poison ivy, 79

Potato raw: burns, 56; insect stings, bites, 75

Powders, 44

Prayer, 29–31, *30*; broken heart, 180; depression, 170; fright, 167, 168–69; house cleansing, 177; for spiritual illness, 158–59

Pregnancy. *See* Childbirth

Premenstrual syndrome (PMS), 107–8

Prostate: enlargement (BPH), 109–12; massage, 142–46, *144–45*

Psoriasis and eczema, 80

Pulse, 32–33

Pumpkin: seeds, for broken heart, 181; seeds, for prostate enlargement, 110–11; vine leaves, for ringworm, 80–81

Purges: adult, 61–62; child, 66, 121–22

Purslane: backache, 49–50; osteoporosis, 106

Radish leaves, for liver ailments, 78

Red clover: anemia, 46; cuts and scrapes, 63

Relaxing teas, 64, 66

Rice, for diarrhea, 119

Ringworm, 80–81

Ritual and ceremony, 37

Rose: for bleeding, excessive, after childbirth, 96; hibiscus and, lotion, for wrinkles, 89–90, *89*; newborn bath, 124; red, tea for diarrhea, 64, 119

Rosemary: dysmenorrhea, 98; incense for spiritual illness, 162, 171, 174; menopause, 103; PMS, 108

Rosy periwinkle tea for menopause, 103

Rue: broken heart, 180, 181; depression, 170; endometriosis, 98–99; fright (susto), 167, *167*; herbal bath for spiritual illness, 160, 170, 179; holy water and, 175; house cleansing, 177; rub, for fainting, 66

Sadness (*tristeza*). *See* Depression
Sage: burning for spiritual illness, 162, 174; as natural antibiotic for skin infections, 128; swelling, 85–86
Saint-John's-wort, for broken heart, 181
Sarsaparilla. *See* China root
Sastun, 36
Saw palmetto for prostate enlargement, 111
Sciatic nerve pain, 35
Sensitive plant (sleepy head, *xmutz*) for insomnia, 75–76, *76*
Sesame seeds: dry skin, 65; milk vs., and calcium content, 106; osteoporosis, 106; prostate enlargement, 110; Toasted, Salsa, 65
Sexual dysfunction: fright, healing, and, 166–67, *167*; impotency, 112–13, 142; painful intercourse, 106; premature ejaculation, 142
Shoulder stiffness, 35
Sick People Soup, 60
Skin ailments: boils, 122, 123; dry, 64–65; infections, children, 122–23, 127–28; psoriasis and eczema, 80; rashes, infant, 123–24; ringworm, 80–81
Skunk root, for ulcers, 86–87
Sleeplessness in children, 124–25
Soap and brown sugar, for boils, 122
Sore throat, 81–82
Soul loss, 7, 153–56; lost souls of a deceased person, ghosts, unemployed spirits, spirit possession, 185–86
Soul retrieval and shamanic journeying, 31
Soy, phyto-estrogens in, 90
Spanish healing terms, xvii

Spirit guides, 36–37
Spirits and healing 7–12
Spiritual illness, 157–86; lost souls of a deceased person, ghosts, unemployed spirits, spirit possession, 185–86; night terrors and, 157; symptoms, 157–58; three-part treatment, 158–62. *See also* Depression; Envy; Evil eye; Fright; Grief
Stomach complaints, 82–84; abdominal massage for, 146–47; five-minute tummy ache massage for infants and children, 149
Stress and anxiety, 64
Strong back plant (Desmodium): asthma, 48; backache, 49
Styes, 84–85
Sulfur powder (flowers of), aloe and, for ringworm, 81
Sunburn, 18, 55
Sweating for colds and flu, 58
Swelling, 85–86
Swimmer's ear, 120

Tamarind fruit, for morning sickness, 94
Teas: black, for sunburn, 55; headache, 73–74; making, 43; relaxing, 64, 66
Temperature change, effect of, 50; cold, foods and drink, during menstruation, 91; cold, and impotency, 113; increasing body's for colds and flu, 58; stomach complaints and, 82–83
Thyme: ear infections, 120; as natural antibiotic for skin infections, 128
Tinctures, 43
Tomato juice cocktail, for sore throat, 81–82
Toothache, 86

Ulcers, 86–88
Urination, frequent, 142, 143
Uterus: massage, 132–42, *133–35, 138, 139–40*; tipped or prolapsed, 90–91, 101, 132, *133–35*, 135–37

Vaginal steam bath, 33, 92–93, *93*
Vaginitis, 108–9
Varicose veins, 142, 143
Ventosa, 35, *35*
Vervain tea for bronchitis, 53
Vinegar, for swimmer's ear, 120

Warts, 88–89; Plantar, 89
Water: diarrhea and, 119; dry skin, 65; guidelines, 194; prostate health, 143; uterine health, 91
Wild yam: China root, and, for gout, 71; gumbo-limbo and, tea, for psoriasis and eczema, 80; menstrual irregularity, 104; Mexican, cream, for PMS, 107–8; Mexican, tea, for menopause, 103; Mexican, tincture, for PMS, 108
Women: abdominal massage for, 146–47; Maya massage for, 132–42; physical ailments of, 90–109, *see also specific ailments*
Wound powder, 63, 123
Wrinkles, 89–90

Xeno-estrogen, 90

Yarrow for toothache, 86
Yellow dock, detoxing with, 45